# NATURAL HO  S

This book is published

# DISCLAIMER

The advice contained in this material might not be suitable for everyone. The author believes that a natural and holistic approach to health and maintaining the body's natural balance.  This material is written for the express purpose of sharing educational information and scientific research gathered from the studies and experiences of the author, healthcare professionals, scientists, nutritionists and informed health advocates.

The author recognizes that within scientific and medical fields there are widely divergent viewpoints and opinions and therefore it is the reader's responsibility to investigate all aspects of any decision before committing him or herself to any treatment. The author obtained the information from sources she believes to be reliable, but she neither implies nor intends any guarantee of accuracy for specific cases or individuals.

Before beginning any practice relating to health, diet or exercise, it is recommended that you first obtain the consent and advice of a licensed health care professional.  The contents of this e-book are not a replacement for professional advice. Always consult your own Doctor or medical professional before starting any treatment, process or action.

The author assumes no responsibility for the choices you make after your review of the information contained herein and your consultation with a licensed healthcare professional. The author, publisher and distributors particularly disclaim any liability, loss, or risk taken by individuals who directly or indirectly act on the information contained in this e-book.  The author believes the advice presented here is sound, but readers cannot hold the author, publisher and distributors responsible for either the actions they take or the results of those actions.

# IMPORTANT

Please note that although the oils, recipes and remedies presented in this book are known to be the most gentle to Sensitive Skins and scalps. As with any natural substance some oils such as thyme can in some individuals cause mild irritation on rare occasions and some oils should NOT be used at all while pregnant – It is recommended that as a precaution you should patch test all oils/formulas before application to skin.

# TABLE OF CONTENTS

# 1. WHY WE BUY SKIN CARE PRODUCTS

We were all born with beautiful baby soft skin but it's no secret that age, diet, lifestyle, sun, stress and illness all take their toll over the years.

We all want to feel good and maintain a youthful healthy glow if we can. To do this most of us include a skincare routine of some sort (even if its soap and water) in our daily routine.

For those of us that buy commercially manufactured skincare products, the fact is that we have been conditioned into treating our skin and scalp on a daily basis with a chemical cocktail of ingredients. These ingredients are designed to keep products fresh, make them smell nice and appear commercially presentable. (Have you noticed how most skin creams are pearly white or unnaturally colored). It is a medically recognized fact that our body absorbs significant amounts of what we put on our skin. Many people have sensitivities to preservatives and other ingredients commonly used in skin care products.

Marketing companies are paid to tell us about the positive effects of their products e.g. "contains AHA fruit oils" but are obviously not going to mention any of the potential hazards in some of the chemical ingredients. Most of the time you'll find it's the petroleum or chemical based ingredients added to products that may be silently damaging our scalp, hair, skin and eyes.

Even some natural labelled products contain synthetic ingredients to keep them in a stable condition so they stay fresh on store shelves. An example is, Lauramide dea, part natural but also part synthetic, which is used to build up a lather that is not only drying but can cause itching and dermatitis. Unfortunately many synthetically processed products are often disguised with "natural or organic sounding names".

Other nasty ingredients in foaming washes to look out for are Sodium lauryl sulfate, Sodium beryl sulfate, and Sodium laureth sulphate (SLS). (Most often used in shampoos and washes). These can all cause a range of allergic reactions like hair loss, wrinkles, dry flaky skin and rashes.

Consumers are becoming increasingly aware of their buying choices, especially from an ecological and wellbeing point of view. This is why so many people are now looking for natural skin care products that are free of toxins and chemicals, while conserving the environment.

By talking about this here, my intent is not to stand on my (organic pesticide and chemical free) soap box and make you uncomfortable - but simply to acknowledge that people are justifiably more aware and concerned about what they are applying to their skin and know that what they read on a product label when buying products is not necessarily clear and transparent.

I am not saying don't use commercially made products – but rather pointing out that knowing what to look for for means you can make an educated decision before paying for skin care products.

What you will discover through reading and using this book is that NONE of the recipes in this book contain anything even remotely synthetic or potentially harmful but instead contain the highly beneficial and active ingredients you'll find in top of the line beauty products.

By sharing the information and recipes in this book you can use natural ingredients to enjoy all the benefits skin care companies proclaim to offer for your skin and more for a fraction of the cost and in an easy hassle free way.

Because ingredients are fresh, they have a much greater "potency" than heat processed, preservative loaded store bought products.

You may be wondering if you can still use natural preservatives to keep your recipes fresh? The answer is yes, however they won't keep as long and do lose some of their benefits over time.

This book will give you the tools and knowledge to make your own custom made to suit your skin beauty products at home using every day ingredients to nourish, feed, repair and rejuvenate skin.

# 2. YOUR SKIN: HOW TO KEEP IT LOOKING GOOD

Your skin is uniquely yours – with all it's unique beauty and imperfections!  No matter how other people see our skin, we usually have our own likes and dislikes or opinions about how WE see it.

Generally skin is classified into the four most common skin type categories used by the cosmetics industry including:

**Normal Skin** (no apparent signs of oily or dry areas)

**Oily Skin** (shine appears all over skin, no dry areas at all)

**Dry Skin** (flaking can appear, no oily areas at all, skin feels tight)

**Combination Skin** (oily, typically in the central part of the face, and dry or normal areas elsewhere)

Whether we classify ourselves into one of these categories (or more realistically a combination of several from oily, dry, blemished or a variety of combinations of skin types) we all want to know how to care for our skin in the best way.

The fact is that most of us have something we want to correct or alleviate and this sometimes means we don't feel as good about our skin as we'd like to.  We want to know what to apply to make our skin look and feel as good as it can.

We usually use the following genres of skin care products to help us do this.

**CLEANSING BARS, CREAMS OR FOAMING CLEANSERS**

**MAKE UP REMOVERS**

**TONERS**

**SCRUBS**

**MOISTURIZERS**

**MASKS**

**TREATMENTS LIKE SERUMS FOR ANTI - AGING**

**EYE CREAMS (WRINKLES, DARK CIRCLES AND TIGHTENING)**

**TREATMENTS FOR ACNE**

**TREATMENTS FOR SPOTS AND SCARRING**

These products contain a whole range of ingredients that are added with specific benefits for your skin from cleansing to moisturizing to treating blemishes.

These ingredients help your skin stay clean, retain or add moisture, exfoliate & remove dead skin cells, encourage new cell growth, whiten, lighten or smooth and more.

How they do this is by using a variety of "active" additives, some natural - some not, some expensive – others cost very little.

Many of these ingredients are derived from plant sources like herbs or extracts or from compounds that attract moisture.

In the next chapter you'll read about what these do so you have an idea of how the recipes in this book will work to nourish and improve your skins appearance and overall wellbeing.

# 3. ACTIVE INGREDIENTS: WHAT THEY DO FOR SKIN

Here's some of the terminology you've probably heard, seen or read in advertising or on the labels of your beauty products.

## ALPHA HYDROXY ACIDS (AHA'S)

These are fruit acids naturally derived from fruit extracts. They slough off dead skin cells to reveal younger more youthful looking skin. As we age our skins renewal process slows down and these help to replace that process giving your skin a younger appearance.

## ANTIOXIDANTS

Ingredients that contain vitamin A, C end E, green tea, copper, grapeseed, and kinetin help skin by neutralizing or scavenging free radicals which are molecules that destroy skin cells.

## BETA-HYDROXY ACIDS

These work in a similar way as AHA's but are less potent so therefore less irritating to skin. The most common and well known one is Salicylic acid which is used in acne treatments and dandruff shampoos.

## BOTANICALS

Ingredients from a naturally derived source (usually plants) believed for centuries to have healing or regenerating powers for the skin. Examples are Aloe Vera, ginko and ginseng.

## COENZYME Q10

This is a nutrient found in every cell of our body known to be a powerful wrinkle buster.

## ESSENTIAL OILS

Most commonly used in aromatherapy to scent products but also as complimentary and healing or regenerating active ingredients in skin care products.

## EMOLLIENTS

Found in moisturizers these ingredients help protect the skin by reinforcing the lower moisture barrier deep in the lower epidermis of the skin. Natural emollients include:

Apricot Kernel Oil, Avocado Oil, Borage Seed Oil, Evening Primrose Oil, Grape Seed Oil, Hazel Nut Oil, Hemp Seed Oil, Kukui Oil, Macadamia Nut Oil, Mango Kernel Butter, Organic, Rose Hip Oil, Organic Sesame Seed Oil, Organic Shea Butter, Organic Sunflower Oil, Safflower Oil, Sesame Seed Oil, Shea Butter, Sunflower Oil, Sweet Almond Oil, Tea Tree Oil, Wheat Germ Oil.

## HYPOALLERGENICS

Ingredients that are low allergy producing ingredients in products.

## MATTIFYERS

Ingredients that soak up oil like cornstarch and witch hazel.

## HUMECTANTS

These are compounds that attract moisture from the air to the skin. Examples are hyaluronic acid, honey, glycerin, glucose & propylene glycol.

## LIPOSOMES

Delivery agents to help skin absorb ingredients deeper.

## RETINOLS

Products high in Vitamin A, for protection against free radicals and some (Retin A and Retinova) dramatically reduce skin damage from the suns rays.

## NON-COMEDOGENICS

Ingredients that don't clog pores and encourage blackheads. The ingredients used in this book are all non-comedogenic.

## ANTI FUNGALS AND ANTI BACTERIALS

Ingredients that combat bacteria and acne related problems. Essential oils like Rosemary, Neem, Tea Tree and others can be added to beauty products to fight bacterial problems.

## HYDROSOLS

Hydrosols are the "left over" by products of making essential oils. Hydrosols in themselves make great toners and have other properties that are very beneficial for skin.

## INFUSIONS OR TEAS

Infusions are herbs or other parts of plants, fruits, skins and barks or teas. They make great toners with soothing, calming & many other properties that are very beneficial for skin. Often used in skincare or hair care recipes to compliment ingredient blends with invigorating, sweetening & other beneficial scents and aromas.

# 4. TOOLS FOR PRODUCT APPLICATION

Here are some useful items you can keep around home to apply to your skin. These are optional items you can use. Most of the time a clean face washcloth will be fine for every day use.

### COTTON BALLS AND SQUARES

For gentle wiping and Exfoliating.

### BAMBOO SCRUB CLOTH

These are great for sloughing off dead skin

### FACIAL BRUSHES

Like the ones used for applying mens shave foam (these do collect bacteria so be aware that you need to replace them regularly if you are using them).

### LOOFAH SPONGE

These are derived from dried gourd and are readily available at stores. Can be used dry for an invigorating body scrub – some say dry brushing with a dry loofah is great for your circulatory system and for your skin in general. Again these need replacing regularly unless dried out on a regular basis because they can attract mold and mildew.

### SEA SPONGE

These make your cleansers go along way and act as very gentle exfoliators so are very popular for applying and removing cleansers and for removing makeup. Again store them carefully and replace regularly so you don't encourage mold growth.

## SYNTHETIC SPONGES

Same as above but some contain mold inhibitors and are generally softer than sea sponge.

## SPRAY BOTTLE

Great for spraying on toners and acne tonics.  Smaller bottles with a fine mist are better for this application.

## TOOTHBRUSH

Yes that's right - a toothbrush is great for scrubbing the soles of your feet and elbows for removing built up skin.

## BANANA SKIN

Save your banana skins for a day or two – can be used to rub cleanser on your face as can kiwi fruit skins which exfoliate your skin well.

# 5. INGREDIENTS & THEIR BENEFITS

Here is a list of vitamins, & other nutrients which are beneficial for skin, hair & nails:

## VITAMIN A

If you are getting an adequate amount of vitamin A from the foods you eat, you shouldn't need to supplement you diet. However, if your vitamin A levels drop even a little below normal, that's when you'll see some skin-related symptoms, including a dry, flaky complexion. The reason for this is that vitamin A is necessary for the maintenance and repair of skin tissue. Without it, you'll see an appreciable difference. Fruits and vegetables are loaded with Vitamin A You can also find vitamin C in butter, eggs, milk, carrots, tomatoes, oily fish, dark green leafy vegetables and apricots making them excellent ingredients for natural skin care recipes.

## VITAMIN B COMPLEX

B vitamin (biotin) is arguably one of if not the most important vitamin for skin. It is a nutrient that forms the basis of all skin, nail, and hair cells. Without adequate amounts, you may see signs of dermatitis (an itchy, scaly skin condition) and even hair loss. If you are deficient in this Vitamin you skin will be one of the first indicators that you are lacking in this vitamin. Generally your body makes more than enough biotin, but the nutrient is also present in many foods, including bananas, eggs, oatmeal, and rice. B complex creams will give you a healthy glow while plumping out and renewing your complexion. Vitamin B complex is found in milk, eggs, wholegrain cereals, bread, wheat germs, nuts, soy beans and tofu, poultry, fish, and meats. Other excellent sources of vitamin B-6 include bananas, potatoes and spinach.

## VITAMIN C

This among the most important new dermatologic discoveries when it comes to combating the effects of sun exposure.  This is because vitamin C is a very potent free radical scavenger and protects against the destruction of collagen and elastin, the fibers that support skin structure which cause wrinkles and other signs of aging.  Vitamin C supplements in your diet help to combat free radicals but are also beneficial applied topically to your skin.  You can also find high concentrations of vitamin C in many essential oils. Foods rich in vitamin C include Blackcurrant, green peppers, citrus fruits, bananas, avocados, artichokes and leafy green vegetables like spinach and silverbeet.

## VITAMIN D

Vitamin D is also a powerful natural vitamin that protects you from free radicals especially from ultraviolet rays and does wonders for your skin. Found in fish liver oils, oily fish, milk and eggs. Also derived from sun exposure.

## VITAMIN E

This is another potent antioxidant that helps reduce the harmful effects of the sun on the skin.  Supplementing your diet with 400 units of vitamin E daily may help to reduce the risk of sun damage to cells and reduce the production of cancer causing cells.   There are studies that show that when vitamins E and A are consumed together, a 70% reduction in basal cell carcinoma, one of the most common forms of skin cancer can e noted.  Vitamin E is also great for reducing wrinkles and make your skin look and feel smoother.  Vitamin E is found in wheat germ, peanuts, vegetable oils, pulses, green leafy vegetables.

## VITAMIN K

Vitamin K can reduce under eye circles and bruises. When combined with vitamin A in a cream, mask or serum, vitamin K can be more effective for reducing the appearance of under eye dark circles.

# MINERALS, OILS & ACIDS BENEFICIAL FOR SKIN

## NUTRITION

Most health experts agree that the majority of us don't need to supplement our mineral intake especially if you drink spring water, which often contains natural quantities of important minerals. Studies have shown that rinsing your face with mineral water can help reduce many common skin irritations, balance your skin's pH and the mineral content may help some skin cells absorb moisture more efficiently.

### SELENIUM

Scientists believe this mineral plays a key role in skin cancer prevention. Taken in supplement form or in a cream, it protects skin from sun damage. If you like to spend any time in the sun, selenium could reduce your chance of burning, lowering your risk of skin cancer. The best dietary sources of selenium include whole-grain cereals, seafood, garlic, and eggs.

## COPPER

Another important mineral for skin is copper. Together with vitamin C and the mineral zinc, copper assists in the development of elastin, the fibers that support the foundation skin structure. Topical applications of copper-rich creams can help to firm the skin and help restore skins elasticity.

## ZINC

Another important mineral for skin is zinc, especially if you have acne. Sometimes acne can be a symptom of a zinc deficiency. Whether taken internally or applied topically, zinc works to clear skin by reducing oil production and can be effective for controlling the formation of acne as well as healing existing acne. Food sources of zinc include oysters, lean meat, and poultry.

## ALPHA-LIPOIC ACID

Another powerful antioxidant, far more potent that vitamin C or E, alpha-lipoic acid is great for aging skin. What is so unique about ALA is its ability to penetrate both oil and water, benefitting skin cells from both the inside and the outside of the body.

It's known to neutralize skin cell damage caused by free radicals repairing damage to skin's DNA, thus reducing the risk of cancer. It can also aid to help other vitamins work more effectively to rebuild skin cells damaged by environmental damage from smoke and pollution. You can supplement your diet with alpha-lipoic acid capsules or alternatively use creams, masks and oil blends that contain ALA antioxidants.

## ALPHA HYDROXY ACIDS

Alpha hydroxy acids are found in many skin care products including moisturizers, cleansers, serums, eye creams, sunscreen, and foundations. They are excellent for exfoliating and renewing skin by dissolving dead skin cells and encouraging new cell growth.

## DMAE

Another powerful antioxidant, this nutrient offers one of the strongest defenses against free radicals. It works mostly by neutralizing the ability of free radicals to harm skin cells. DMAE is especially effective against age spots and can be taken in supplements and in topical creams.

## HYALURONIC ACID

Made by the body, this nutrient's main job is to lubricate joints so that knees, elbows, fingers, and toes all move smoothly and easily. The same can be said of HA for keeping skin looking smoother and younger. Hyaluronic acid also can hold up to 1,000 times its weight in water, binding more moisture to each skin cell. Many top of the line skin care creams contain HA and as the body does not manufacture it, it's highly beneficial for skin when added to skin care products.

# ESSENTIAL FATTY ACIDS (EFAS)

If your skin is dry, prone to inflammation, and you have frequent breakouts of white heads and black heads, you could be lacking essential fatty acids. These are nutrients that are crucial to the production of skin's natural oil barrier. These are "good oils" that contain beneficial balancing and nourishing benefits for skin. You can find EFA's mainly in foods like cold-water fish, like salmon, sardines, and mackerel, flaxseed, and flax and safflower oils. Taking supplements including fish oil capsules or evening primrose oil may help keep your skin smoother and younger-looking. Flaxseed oil, walnuts and almonds are also a good source of omega-3 fatty acids.

## CALCIUM

Found in cheese, nuts, eggs, milk, yogurt, sardines, root vegetables. A good source of calcium and other beneficial nutrients are found in coconut water Consumed and/or applied 2 – 3 times a week, it is good for your skin, digestive system and hair.

## IODINE

Great for your general wellbeing, found in seafood, dried kelp, iodized salt.

## IRON

Found in spinach, cockles, liver, kidneys, pulses, lentils, beans, peas, dried fruit. Keeps color in your complexion and helps your skin glow.

## PROTEIN

Many legumes such as beans and vegetables are high in protein content. Lean meat like fish, chicken, eggs, Yogurt, cheese, sunflower seeds and soy products are good sources of protein also.

## SULFUR

Topical sulfur is most commonly used to treat skin-related conditions. Sulfur has several potential uses for skin care including topical sulfur ointments for treating acne, seborrheic dermatitis, rosacea, eczema and dandruff. Sulfur helps reduce skin oiliness & blocked pores.

You can apply sulfur topically to help treat warts, pityriasis versicolor or skin discoloration, hair-follicle infections and shingles, Sulfur assists in shedding excessive skin and fighting bacteria on the skin. Found in eggs, meat, cheese, dairy products, fish, garlic, onions, dairy and beans.

# 6. INGREDIENTS & THEIR APPLICATION

These are some of the ingredients you have at your disposal to create recipes with – some are more exotic than others, giving you the choice and a wide range of ingredients to use as alternatives in your recipes.

**INGREDIENTS & THEIR BENEFITS**

**ALMOND MEAL**

Made from: Ground raw (not roasted) almonds

Useful for: Scrubs masks and exfoliants

Benefits for skin: Slightly bleaching and exfoliating

**ALMOND OIL**

Made from: Pressed almonds

Useful for: Moisturizing lotions, creams, balms.  Can be used straight as a moisturizer on its own or as a carrier base for essential oils.

Benefits for skin: High fatty acid concentration so very moisturizing and great for itchy inflamed skin

**ALOE VERA**

Made from: Aloe plant

Useful for: Fresh gel from plant or bottled juice

Benefits for skin: Mild astringent, healing and soothes irritation plus helps restore the skins pH balance

## ANISE SEED OIL

Made from: Essential oil of anise

Useful for: A warming stimulating oil that is used for scenting skin care products and lip balms

Benefits for skin: Fragrance

Cautions: Avoid using if pregnant or epileptic and can irritate Sensitive Skin

## APPLE

Made from: Fresh, pureed or juice

Useful for: Contains renewing AHA (malic) acid and is a mild astringent

Benefits for skin: Gentle exfoliating properties, good for sensitive and acneic skin

Cautions: Avoid using on sunburned or wind burnt skin

## APPLE CIDER VINEGAR

Made from: Apples raw

Useful for: Gently exfoliating and soothing, relieves itchy skin and scalp

Benefits for skin: Exfoliating, balance pH

Cautions: Avoid using on sunburned or wind burnt skin

APRICOT KERNEL OIL

Made from: Essential oil of anise

Useful for: A warming stimulating oil that is used for scenting skin care products and lip balms

Benefits for skin: Fragrance, penetrates into skin well, moisturizing, delivers other ingredients deep into skin.

## APRICOTS RAW

Made from: Apricots

Useful for: Ground seeds are exfoliating and flesh contains fruit acids

Benefits for skin: Exfoliating, sulfur content and aha acids help exfoliate & lift off dead skin cells

Cautions: Avoid using ground seeds on irritated skin

## ARGAN OIL

Made from: Argan tree kernels

Useful for: Oil blends

Benefits for skin: Argan oil offer some of the best anti-wrinkle properties and is also useful for scars

## ARROWROOT

Made from: Arrowroot ground and powdered

Useful for: Powders

Benefits for skin: Use like talcum powder

## AVOCADO

Made from: Avocado (oil and pulp)

Useful for: Creams, lotions, face masks.

Benefits for skin: Penetrates skin well and contains fatty acids as well as vitamins A, B1, B2, D and E for dry skin.  It is protective so is great for people who love to be outdoors and prevents moisture evaporation.

## ARGAN OIL

Made from: Argan nuts

Useful for: Hair, skin and scalp moisturizer and conditioner

Benefits for skin: Moisturizer topically applied will not only help to soften up your skin, but it also helps with ski problems. The polyunsaturated fatty acids as well as the vitamin E are good antioxidants which promote oxygenation within the cells neutralizing adverse effects of free radicals. Protective and renewing. Good penetration properties.

## BAKING SODA

Made from: Mineral compound

Useful for: Bath additive, stings and bite tinctures and deodorants

Benefits for skin: Softening & alkalizing skin, soothes bites, stings and also helps deodorize smells (especially feet and underarms)

## BANANA

Made from: Bananas fresh

Useful for: Face masks

Benefits for skin: Non abrasive moisturizing mask and exfoliant.

Tightens skin and is good for all skin types especially normal and dry.

## BASIL (SWEET)

Made from: Essential oil

Useful for: Great for hair, scalp and stimulating hair growth

Benefits for skin: Like Rosemary oil it has hair growth stimulating properties and is antibacterial so helps with scalp pimples and irritation

Cautions: Avoid if you are pregnant or epileptic

## BERGAMOT

Made from: Essential oil (orange citrus scented)

Useful for: Creams, lotions and balms for acne prone skin & relaxation

Benefits for skin: Great for acne and boils

Cautions: Avoid while pregnant or epileptic and avoid too much sun

## BEESWAX

Made from: Bees wax

Useful for: Emollient and humectant in crams and lotions

Benefits for skin: Helps keep moisture in - used as a "binding agent" in skin creams

## BLACKBERRY OR RASPBERRY

Made from: Blackberries or raspberries

Useful for: Astringent for normal to oily skin

Benefits for skin: Balancing oily or normal skin.  Berries are high in vitamins and antioxidants

## BROWN SUGAR

Made from: Sugar cane

Useful for: Scrubs and masks

Benefits for skin: Contains fruit (glycolic) acids so great for exfoliating dead skin cells, also a humectant and great for making yummy moisturizing face and body scrubs especially when combined with honey and fruits

## CASTOR OIL

Made from: Made from castor oil plant

Useful for: Lip gloss, lipsticks and on cracked heels etc

Benefits for skin: Very moisturizing glossy agent in makeup

## CALENDULA

Made from: Flower petals (an essential oil)

Useful for: Healing anti inflammatory balms & kids, similar to chamomile

Benefits for skin: Great for windblown chapped lips & skin.  Especially soothing for sensitive or damaged skin

### CALOPHYLLUM OIL

Made from: Seeds of a native Tahitian tree

Useful for: Oils blends for analgesic, anti inflammatory purposes for scarring, burns, chapped skin, eczema and psoriasis

Benefits for skin: Soothing calming healing oil

### CARROT SEED OIL

Made from: Carrot seeds

Useful for: Facial serums, eye treatment creams

Benefits for skin: Saggy wrinkled sun damaged skin.  High in vitamin A so good for all skin types.  Regenerating, rejuvenating essential oil that stimulates circulation and aids in repairing and toning the skin while increasing skin elasticity, helping reduce wrinkles.

Cautions: Avoid while pregnant or epileptic and avoid too much sun

### CEDARWOOD

Made from: Essential oil of cedar

Useful for: Insect repellent

Benefits for skin: Biting insect deterrent

## CHAMOMILE (GERMAN)

Made from: Chamomile flowers (tea and essential oil)

Useful for: Calming irritated skin and itching

Benefits for skin: Calms babies rashes, toning skin and lightening hair. Good for normal or dry skin.  Chamomile is great for Inflammation and is renowned for its cosmetic and conditioning benefits to skin and hair. It makes a great conditioner for hair moreover enhances color in blond and red hair.  Splash your face with chamomile tea a few times a week to add a glow to your skin.

## CHOCOLATE

Made from: Cocoa beans

Useful for: Creams butters, lotions.

Benefits for skin: Smells delicious (think chocolate & vanilla) and is moisturizing for skin

## CINNAMON

Made from: Cinnamon bark

Useful for: Fragrance for balms and lotions

Benefits for skin: Smells nice but can be irritating

## CITRONELLA

Made from: Essential oil of citrus

Useful for: Natural insect repellent

Benefits for skin: Biting insect deterrent

## COSMETIC CLAYS (WHITE GREEN AND RED)

Made from: Mineral earth

Useful for: Masks, cleansing and exfoliating

Benefits for skin: High in minerals and draws toxins, excess oils and dirt from the skin. Great for oily problematic skin.

White Clay is good for environmentally damaged sensitive & mature skins (not dry skin).

Green Clay is good for oily and combination or acneic skin because it reduces sebum or oils.

Red Clay is great for cleansing and toning of general skin types

## COCOA BUTTER

Made from: Cocoa beans

Useful for: Creams butters, lotions.

Benefits for skin: Smells delicious (think chocolate & vanilla) and is moisturizing for skin

## COCONUT OIL OR MILK

Made from: Coconuts

Useful for: An emollient and used in creams, lotions and on its own to penetrate skin

Benefits for skin: Softening and moisturizing

## STARFLOWER (BORAGE) OIL

Made from: Starflower plant

Useful for: Anti ageing moisturizing serum

Benefits for skin: Very moisturizing anti ageing smoothing oil

## CUCUMBER

Made from: Cucumber plant

Useful for: Fresh facial masks & toners

Benefits for skin: Astringent soothing with mild whitening effect

## EGG WHITES

Made from: Eggs separated

Useful for: Cleansers, face masks and tightening serums

Benefits for skin: Tightening, lightening effect, good for firming sagging skin

## ELDER FLOWER

Made from: Flowers

Useful for: Soothing cleanser/toner

Benefits for skin: Soothing for eye and skin irritation

## EPSON SALTS (MAGNESIUM SULPHATE)

Made from: Magnesium sulphate

Useful for: Aches and pain relief in the bath for sore muscles

Benefits for skin: Drying but relaxing for muscles and a clenched jaw

Cautions: Not good for irritated or dry skin but good to relax aches and pains

## EUCALYPTUS

Made from: Essential oil of Eucalyptus trees

Useful for: Acne related facial masks and clearing sinus passages

Benefits for skin: Antiseptic, antibacterial and sinus clearing. Cools the skin (tingling sensation)

## EGGPLANT OR AUBERGINE

Made from: Eggplant plant

Useful for: Facial mask base for Sensitive Skin

Benefits for skin: Vitamins B, A, E and antioxidant properties

## EMU OIL

Made from: Emu oil

Useful for: Creams, on its own, in blends and face masks

Benefits for skin: Hypoallergenic, anti inflammatory, antibacterial and moisturizing. Also good for scars and stretch marks

## EVENING PRIMROSE OIL

Made from: Evening primrose pressed oil

Useful for: Serums, moisturizers and straight application. Dietary supplement

Benefits for skin: Hormone balancing, great for reducing acne, breakouts and skin smoothing. Balances skin sebum so you have the right amount of oil production in your skin.

## FENNEL

Made from: Essential oil

Useful for: Toning, steaming, cleansers and toners.  Makes a good foot scrub and body cleanser too

Benefits for skin: Deodorizing, moisturizing and refreshingly sweet

## FIGS

Made from: Pulp of fig fruit

Useful for: Facial masks

Benefits for skin: Loaded with Vitamin C and natural fruit acids, gentle exfoliator when seeds left in mashed and rubbed over skin

## FISH OILS

Made from: Fish oil and packaged in capsules

Useful for: Meals and dietary supplement

Benefits for skin: Omega 3 Vitamin B oils are great for all aspects of skincare.  Moisturizing, plumping and making your skin glow.

## FRANKINCENSE

Made from: Essential oil

Useful for: Addition to moisturizers, lotions & carrier oils applied to skin

Benefits for skin: For tired, sagging, blemished skin.  Helps heal skin and is great to add to a blend for mature, acneic or mature skin. Encourages skin cell growth.

## GOTU KOLA (BRAHMI)

Made from: Gotu Kola leaves

Useful for: Removes excess oils from skin and hair

Benefits for skin: Balancing skin & improving mental function/memory

## GUAVA

Made from: Guava berries

Useful for: Facial masks

Benefits for skin: Guava is effective for skin whitening and as natural bleach for the skin. Also has high vitamin & antioxidant properties.

## GRAPE SEED OIL

Made from: Grape seeds pressed oil

Useful for: Add to carrier base oils, moisturizers, masks

Benefits for skin: Moisturizing, penetrating (takes ingredients deep into skin) protective. Rich in antioxidants and OPCs, otherwise known as oligomeric proanthocyanidin complexes.  A little too greasy for very oily skin.

## GERANIUM

Made from: Geranium flowers and plant oil

Useful for: Facial masks, sebums and moisturizers

Benefits for skin: Repairs damaged exposed skin and helps balance sebum production

## GINGER

Made from: Ginger root (fresh or oil)

Useful for: Facial masks and scrubs

Benefits for skin: Stimulates circulation and enlivens the skin.  Renews cells and gives a tingling sensation

## HAZELNUTS

Made from: Hazelnuts

Useful for: Facial masks and scrubs

Benefits for skin: Exfoliating and moisturizing

## HYDROSOLS (FLOWER WATERS)

Made from: Byproduct of essential oil distillation process

Useful for: Spray spritzing bottles, toners and for hydration. Can be added to moisturizers and toners.

Benefits for skin: They are generally very gentle and soft for your skin

There are many hydrosols listed below:

Chamomile: Soothing calming floral type fragrance, good for sensitive irritated weathered or mature skins.

**Clary sage:** Perfect for dry and aging skin, clary sage relieves skin problems associated with hormone issues and menopause.

**Rose:** Balancing astringent properties, again good for sensitive irritated or environmentally damaged skin.

**Lavender:** An astringent, calming and has antiseptic qualities so its good for acneic or irritated skin and wind or sunburnt skin.

**Neroli:** Freshly fragranced (orange blossoms) good for sensitive irritated or environmentally damaged skin as well as acneic or irritated and wind or sunburnt skin.

## JOJOBA OIL

Made from: Jojoba seeds

Useful for: On its own its a great moisturizer but can be added to moisturizers, creams or as a base oil to add other essential oils to.

Benefits for skin: Moisturizing, great for hair skin and nails. Mimics skins sebum and helps deliver other ingredients in skin care products deep into the skin.

## JUNIPER OIL

Made from: Juniper berries

Useful for: Creams, lotions and oils

Benefits for skin: Balances oily and acneic skin as well as cellulite

Cautions: Avoid if pregnant epileptic and can irritate skin if too concentrated

## KARANJA OIL

Made from: Bark of tree related to Neem oil

Useful for: Adding to base oils and creams and insect repellants

Benefits for skin: Relief for itching, wounds, antibacterial and insect repelling. Anti bacterial and anti fungal

## KIWI FRUIT

Made from: Kiwi fruit (Chinese gooseberry)

Useful for: Facial masks

Benefits for skin: AHA's great for exfoliating dead skin cells and you can even use the rough skin before peeling as a rub for feet and elbows etc

## LANOLIN

Made from: Sheep gland secretion

Useful for: Emollient and waxy type moisturizer ingredient

Benefits for skin: Good for dry skin and is an emulsifier (absorbs moisture)

## LAVENDER OIL OR FRESH LEAVES

Made from: Essential oil or leaves & flowers

Useful for: teas and infusions or added to base oils and moisturizers, lotions, creams and masks

Benefits for skin: Calming for sensitive irritated or itchy skin. Lavender is great in cleansers and toners for acneic skin also

## MACADAMIAS

Made from: Macadamia nuts

Useful for: Facial masks and oil blends

Benefits for skin: Soothing, moisturizing and mimics skins sebum

## MANUKA OIL

Made from: Manuka tree

Useful for: Creams butters, lotions, acne masks

Benefits for skin: Has good antibacterial, antifungal, and anti-inflammatory properties providing an effective natural acne treatment

## MELONS

Made from: Rock melon (cantelope), watermelon and others

Useful for: Refreshing masks and spritzers

Beneficial for: Vitamins and moisture. Melons also contain AHAs to gently exfoliate your skin and slough off dead skin cells

## MILK PRODUCTS POWDERED AND FRESH

Made from: Dairy

Useful for: Facial masks, cleansers

Benefits for skin: Contain lactic acids and Vitamins to moisturize and gently exfoliate skin

## MINT

Made from: Mint leaves

Useful for: Infusion & masks

Benefits for skin: Refreshing and good for oily skin

## MYRHH

Made from: A tree resin

Useful for: Facial masks and lotions

Benefits for skin: Antiseptic, antibacterial & anti fungal. Great for infections too. Balances and adds hydration. Aids with removal of toxins and promotes tissue repair.

## NEEM OIL

Made from: Bark of Neem tree

Useful for: Adding to base oils and creams and insect repellants

Benefits for skin: Relief for itching, wounds, antibacterial and insect repelling. Antibacterial and anti fungal. Also has a low SPF but smells very strong so not popular as a sunscreen

## NEROLI OIL

Made from: Blossom of the bitter orange tree

Useful for: Masks and oil blends

Benefits for skin: Stimulates cells and aids in repairing broken capillaries. Increases elasticity of mature skin so good for wrinkles and sagging skin.

## OATMEAL

Made from: Oats ground and/or flaked

Useful for: Scrubs, exfoliators, strained liquid for relief from itching

Benefits for skin: Soothing for itchy irritated skin from bites or plant reactions and dry Sensitive Skin

## OLIVE OIL (EXTRA VIRGIN)

Made from: Olive tree pressed oil

Useful for: Facial masks, moisturizing blends of oils, cleansers and scarring blends

Benefits for skin: Moisturizing, scarring, stretch marks, contains loads of vitamins and minerals for skin and hair

## ORANGE (OIL OR FRESH)

Made from: Orange juice, rind (peel), flesh and oil from skin

Useful for: Facial masks, cleansers, toners, creams and lotions (oil)

Benefits for skin: Astringent, antioxidant. Good for oily skin and cellulite

Cautions: Not recommended if pregnant, epileptic or after sun exposure

## PAPAYA & PAW PAW

Made from: Payaya or Paw Paw fruit

Useful for: Cleansers, facial masks as exfoliators.

Benefits for skin: Papaya and paw paw are high in protein digesting enzymes (papain) and fruits acids to slough off dead skin cells and stimulate new cell growth. Papaya in contains natural alpha hydroxy acids (AHAs) and papain, which is an enzyme that works well for exfoliating the skin and stimulating new cell production. Papaya is beneficial for preventative or restorative skin care, helps to heal acne, reduce wrinkles, restore and rejuvenate skin. Its also loaded with: Vitamin A accelerating the formation of new skin cell and Vitamin C, which is an anti-oxidant and beta-carotene, which protects the skin and promotes the skins elasticity.

Papaya is something I use all the time adding it to many other masks in this book.

## PARSLEY (FRESH OR OIL)

Made from: Parsley leaf or oil

Useful for: Infusions, facial masks, moisturizers and lotions

Benefits for skin: Astringent, soothing and healing especially for skin with acne, psoriasis, eczema. Also used regularly in oil blended form can reduce red veins

## PATCHOULI

Made from: Essential oil

Useful for: Facial masks and oil blends or serums

Benefits for skin: Promotes and stimulates new cell growth. Calms red or inflamed skin.

## PEACH

Made from: Fresh pulp

Useful for: Facial masks and cleansers

Benefits for skin: Moisturizing for dry skin. Very high in nutrients and vitamins

## PEPPERMINT

Made from: Peppermint leaves or oil

Useful in: Cleansers, facial masks and scrubs

Benefits for skin: Cooling stimulating and refreshing. Good for oily or normal, combination and acneic skin. Also good for foot scrubs as its deodorizing

## PINEAPPLE

Made from: Pineapple fruit

Useful for: Cleansers, facial masks as exfoliators

Benefits for skin: Pineapple is high in protein digesting enzymes (bromelain) and fruits acids to slough off dead skin cells and stimulate new cell growth. Brightening lightening and is a deep cleanser

## PUMPKIN

Made from: Pumpkin kernels or flesh pulp

Useful for: Facial masks and scrubs

Benefits for skin: Good for all skin types, especially environmentally damaged or Sensitive Skin. High in Vitamin A C and Zinc. Soothes skin and assists other mask ingredients to absorb deeper into the skin.

## ROSE OR ROSE OTTO (OIL)

Made from: Flower petals

Useful for: Hydrosols, spritzers, cleansers, toners, moisturizing lotions and creams as well as in oil blends.

Benefits for skin: Astringent, great for mature or damaged skins and regenerates and renews cells. Excellent hydration properties and promotes skins elasticity

## ROSE HIP (BOIS DE ROSE)

Made from: Rose hip seeds

Useful for: Facial masks, moisturizers, oil blends especially

Benefits for skin: Loaded with fatty acids so has powerful anti aging and repairing qualities for damaged lackluster skin.  Very healing, softening and rejuvenating. Rich in omega acids to rejuvenate aged and sun-damaged skin, and penetrates the skin quickly.

### ROSEMARY (OIL OR LEAVES)

Made from: Rosemary oil or leaves

Useful for: Scrubs, lotions, oil blends and facial masks

Benefits for skin: Antiseptic and antibacterial, good for itching, acne and problem skin.  Refreshing, stimulates skin and circulation, it's mildly astringent so is also good for oily skin.

### SANDALWOOD

Made from: Sandalwood tree oil

Useful for: Facial Masks and oil blends

Benefits for skin: Balancing and nourishing

### SAGE

Made from: Sage leaves or oil

Useful for: Facial masks, infusions and teas.

Benefits for skin: Antibacterial for acneic and oily, combination and normal skin

### SEA SALT (MINERAL SALTS)

Made from: Salt flats or sea salt

Useful for: Rubs, scrubs and exfoliators

Benefits for skin: Drying and healing for acne and other "weepy" sores

Cautions:  Very drying so not good for all over use on face or body

## SESAME OIL

Made from: Sesame seeds

Useful for: Scrubs, exfoliators, facial masks, moisturizers and healing moisturizing oil blends

Benefits for skin: Loaded with vitamins A and E so good for repairing damaged skin and has some SPF protection. Normal to dry skin benefits best from this oil and penetrates deep into skin tissues.

## SHEA BUTTER

Made from: Karite tree nuts

Useful for: Facial masks, creams, lotions and on its own

Benefits for skin: Emollient so absorbs water and other liquids well. Very moisturizing.

## SOYBEAN OIL

Made from: Soy beans

Useful for: Base oil for blends and as a base for insect repellant

Benefits for skin: Good base moisturizer

## STRAWBERRIES

Made from: Strawberries

Useful for: Facial masks, infusions, cleansers

Benefits for skin: Good for normal to oily skin, exfoliating as it contains fruit acids

## STARFLOWER (BORAGE) OIL

Made from: Starflower plant

Useful for: Anti ageing moisturizing serum, oil from capsules can be used direct as a treatment serum

Benefits for skin: Very moisturizing anti ageing smoothing oil

**SUNFLOWER SEEDS GROUND**

Made from: Ground sunflower seeds

Useful for: Scrubs, facial masks.

Benefits for skin: High in essential fatty acids, nutrients, and has emollient properties to mixes well with other ingredients to form a moisturizing face mask base

**SUNFLOWER OIL**

Made from: Sunflower seeds pressed

Useful for: Base oil for blends and as a base for moisturizers, creams and lotions also

Benefits for skin: Good base moisturizer as it's high in fatty acids and also as an antioxidant because of the high levels of A, D and E it contains. Penetrates well into skin and can be a little heavy for oily skins

**TEA TREE (MELALEUCA OIL) OR MANUKA OIL**

Made from: Tea tree

Useful for: Facial masks, cleansers, acne treatments, scrubs, moisturizers, in base oils and lotions

Benefits for skin: Numerous benefits for problematic or acneic skin. Antibacterial, anti fungal and anti viral as well. Great for cuts, sores, grazes and in insect repellants

**THYME**

Made from: Thyme leaves or essential oil

Useful for: Facial masks, cleansers, acne treatments, scrubs, moisturizers, in base oils and lotions

Benefits for skin: Problematic or acneic skin and antibacterial, anti fungal skins. Good from treating rashes and itching

## UMF ACTIVE MANUKA HONEY

Made from: Active Manuka Honey (New Zealand)

Useful for: Creams butters, lotions, acne masks

Benefits for skin: Moisturizing, healing properties. Has good antibacterial, antifungal, and anti-inflammatory properties providing an effective natural acne treatment. Available from health stores - has been considered a remedy for many health conditions since ancient times. Active Manuka Honey is Apply to wounds or sores for healing.

## VANILLA

Made from: Vanilla beans

Useful for: Fragrancing recipes

Benefits for skin: Nothing notable - just smells lovely

## VITAMIN E OIL

Made from: Vitamin E capsules

Useful for: Addition to base oils and moisturizers, lotions and creams. Has preserving qualities. Also use in face masks our on its own

Benefits for skin: Antioxidant

## WALNUT HUSKS

Made from: Ground walnut shells

Useful for: Harsh Exfoliating scrubs

Benefits for skin: Good for foot scrubs and elbows - too harsh for facial skin but good for body

## WHEAT GERM

Made from: Fresh wheat germ

Useful for: Facial masks

Benefits for skin: Good for very dry skin, nourishing for Sensitive Skin due to the high fatty acid contact and vitamin content

## YARROW

Made from: Leaves and flowers

Useful for: Infusions and facial masks

Benefits for skin: Good for oily acneic problem skin or cuts and grazes

## Yogurt

Made from: Animal milk

Useful for: Facial masks, exfoliants and cleansers

Benefits for skin: Moisturizing, contains lactic acid and has a mild bleaching effect on skin.  Good for tender environmentally effected skin (sun sea and wind etc). Also helps to heal damaged skin.

## YAMS/SWEET POTATO

Made from: Sweet potato or yam

Useful for: Good base for facial masks as an alternative to pumpkin or other bases

Benefits for skin: Softening and smoothing

| Wrinkles | Tightening | Stimulating | SPF (Low protection) | Soothing (Irritated Skin) | Repairing | Red Veins | Oily Skin/Blackheads | Moisturizing | Mature Skins | Make Up Removal | Lightening/Brightening | Inflamed Skin (Calming) | Itchy Skin | Healing/Scarring/Damage | Exfoliation (Granule) | Exfoliation (Acids) | Discoloration | Dark Circles/Puffiness | Cooling (Sunburnt Skin) | Insect Repellant | Cleansing | Cellulite | Balancing | Anti-Septic/Anti-Bacterial | Anti-Oxidant | Anti-Inflammatory | Anti-Fungal | Anti-Aging | Age Spots | Acne | Ingredients & Benefits |
|---|---|---|---|---|---|---|---|---|---|---|---|---|---|---|---|---|---|---|---|---|---|---|---|---|---|---|---|---|---|---|---|
|  |  |  |  |  | * |  | * | * |  |  | * |  |  |  | * |  |  |  |  |  |  |  |  |  |  | * |  | * |  | * | Almond Meal |
|  |  |  |  |  | * |  | * | * |  |  |  |  |  |  |  |  |  |  |  |  |  |  |  | * | * | * |  | * |  | * | Almond Oil |
|  |  |  |  |  |  | * |  | * |  |  |  |  |  | * |  |  |  |  |  |  | * |  |  |  | * |  |  |  | * | * | Aloe Vera |
|  |  |  | * |  |  | * |  | * |  |  |  |  |  |  |  |  | * |  |  |  | * |  |  |  | * |  |  |  | * | * | Alpha-Lipoic Acid |
|  |  | * |  |  |  |  |  |  |  |  |  |  |  |  |  |  |  |  |  |  |  |  |  |  |  |  |  |  |  | * | Anise Seed Oil |
| * |  |  |  |  |  |  | * |  |  |  |  |  |  |  |  | * |  |  |  |  | * |  |  |  | * |  |  |  |  | * | Apple |
|  |  |  |  |  | * |  | * | * |  |  |  |  |  | * |  |  |  |  |  |  | * |  | * |  | * |  |  |  |  | * | Apple Cider Vinegar |
| * |  |  |  |  |  |  |  | * |  |  |  |  | * | * |  |  |  |  |  |  | * |  | * |  |  |  |  | * |  |  | Apricot Kernel Oil |
|  |  |  |  |  |  |  |  |  |  | * |  |  |  |  |  | * |  |  |  |  | * |  |  |  | * |  |  |  |  | * | Apricots Raw |
|  |  |  |  |  |  |  |  | * | * |  |  |  |  |  |  |  |  |  |  |  |  |  |  |  | * |  |  |  |  | * | Argan Oil |
|  |  |  |  |  |  |  | * |  |  |  |  |  |  |  |  |  |  |  |  |  |  |  |  |  |  |  |  |  |  | * | Arrowroot |
|  |  |  |  |  |  |  |  |  |  |  |  |  |  |  |  |  |  |  |  |  |  |  |  |  | * |  |  |  |  |  | Aubergine |
| * |  |  |  |  | * |  | * | * |  |  |  |  |  |  |  |  |  |  |  |  |  |  |  |  | * | * |  |  |  |  | Avocado |
|  |  |  |  |  |  |  |  |  |  |  |  |  |  |  | * |  |  |  |  |  |  |  |  | * | * |  |  | * |  | * | Baking Soda |
| * |  | * |  |  | * |  |  | * |  | * |  |  |  |  |  | * |  |  |  |  | * |  |  |  | * |  |  | * |  | * | Alpha-Hydroxy Acid |
| * |  |  |  |  |  |  |  | * |  |  |  |  |  |  |  | * |  |  |  |  | * |  |  |  | * |  |  |  |  |  | Banana |
|  |  |  |  |  |  |  |  |  |  |  |  |  |  |  |  |  |  |  |  |  | * |  |  |  | * |  |  |  |  | * | Basil |
|  |  |  |  |  |  |  |  |  |  |  |  |  |  |  |  |  |  |  |  |  | * |  |  |  | * | * |  |  |  | * | Bergamot |
|  |  |  |  |  |  |  | * | * |  |  |  |  |  |  |  |  |  |  |  |  | * |  |  |  | * | * |  |  |  |  | Berries |
|  |  |  |  |  |  |  | * |  |  |  |  |  |  |  |  | * |  |  |  |  | * |  |  |  |  |  |  |  |  |  | Brown Sugar |
|  |  |  |  | * | * |  |  |  |  |  |  |  | * | * |  |  |  |  |  |  |  |  |  |  |  | * |  |  |  | * | Calendula |
|  |  |  |  | * | * |  |  |  |  |  |  |  |  | * |  |  |  |  |  |  |  |  |  |  |  | * |  |  |  |  | Calophyllum Oil |
| * |  |  |  |  |  |  | * | * |  |  |  |  |  | * |  |  |  |  |  |  |  |  | * | * | * |  |  | * | * | * | Carrot Seed |
|  |  |  |  |  |  |  | * |  |  |  |  |  |  |  |  |  |  |  |  |  |  |  |  |  |  |  |  |  |  |  | Castor Oil |
|  |  |  |  |  |  |  |  |  |  |  |  |  |  |  |  |  |  |  |  |  |  | * |  |  |  |  |  |  |  |  | Cedarwood |
|  |  |  |  | * | * |  |  |  |  |  |  | * | * | * | * |  |  |  |  |  |  |  |  |  | * |  |  |  |  |  | Chamomile |
|  |  |  |  | * |  |  | * |  |  |  |  |  |  |  |  |  |  |  |  |  |  |  |  |  |  |  |  |  |  |  | Chocolate |
| * |  |  |  |  |  |  | * | * |  |  |  |  |  |  |  |  |  |  |  |  |  |  |  |  |  |  |  | * |  |  | Clary Sage |
|  |  |  |  |  |  |  | * | * |  |  |  |  |  |  |  |  |  |  |  |  |  |  |  |  |  |  |  |  |  |  | Cocoa Butter |
|  |  |  |  |  |  |  | * | * |  |  |  |  |  |  |  |  |  |  |  |  |  |  | * | * |  |  |  | * |  |  | Coconut |
|  |  | * |  |  |  | * |  |  |  | * |  |  |  |  |  | * | * |  |  |  | * |  |  |  | * |  |  | * |  | * | Cream |
|  |  | * |  |  |  |  |  |  |  | * |  |  |  |  |  | * | * | * | * |  |  |  | * |  |  |  |  | * | * | * | Cucumber |
| * |  | * |  |  |  | * |  |  |  | * |  |  |  |  |  |  |  |  |  |  | * |  |  |  | * |  |  |  |  | * | Egg Whites |
|  |  |  |  |  |  |  |  |  |  |  |  |  |  | * |  |  |  |  |  |  | * |  | * | * | * |  |  |  |  |  | Elder Flower |
| * |  | * |  |  |  |  |  |  |  |  |  |  |  |  |  |  |  |  | * |  |  |  |  |  |  |  |  |  |  | * | Eucalyptus |
| * |  |  |  |  | * |  | * | * |  | * |  |  |  |  |  |  |  |  |  |  |  |  | * | * |  |  |  | * |  | * | Evening Primrose Oil |
|  |  |  |  |  |  |  |  | * |  |  |  |  |  |  |  |  |  |  |  |  |  |  |  |  |  |  |  |  |  |  | Fennel |
|  |  |  |  |  |  |  |  |  |  |  |  |  |  |  |  | * |  |  |  |  |  |  |  |  | * |  |  |  |  |  | Figs |
| * |  | * |  |  |  |  | * | * |  |  |  |  |  |  |  |  |  |  |  |  |  |  |  |  | * |  |  | * |  | * | Frankincense |
|  |  |  |  |  | * |  |  |  |  |  |  |  |  | * |  |  |  |  |  |  |  |  | * |  |  |  |  |  |  |  | Geranium |
|  | * | * |  |  |  |  |  |  |  |  |  |  |  |  |  |  |  |  |  |  |  |  |  |  |  |  |  | * |  |  | Ginger |
|  |  |  |  |  |  |  | * |  |  |  |  |  |  |  |  |  |  |  |  |  |  |  |  |  |  |  |  |  |  | * | Gotu Kola |
|  |  |  |  |  |  |  | * |  |  |  |  |  |  |  |  |  |  |  |  |  |  | * |  |  |  |  |  | * |  |  | Grape Seed Oil |
|  |  |  |  |  |  |  | * |  |  |  |  |  |  |  |  | * |  |  |  |  | * |  |  |  | * |  |  |  |  |  | Guava |
|  |  |  |  |  |  |  | * |  |  |  |  |  |  | * |  | * |  |  |  |  |  |  |  |  |  |  |  |  |  |  | Hazelnuts |
|  |  |  |  |  | * |  | * | * |  | * |  |  |  | * |  | * |  |  |  |  | * |  |  |  | * | * |  | * |  |  | Honey |
|  |  |  |  |  |  |  | * |  |  |  |  |  |  |  |  |  |  |  |  |  | * |  |  |  | * |  |  | * |  |  | Jojoba Oil |
|  |  |  |  |  |  |  | * |  |  |  |  |  |  |  |  |  |  |  |  |  |  |  | * | * |  |  |  |  |  | * | Juniper |
|  |  |  |  |  |  |  | * |  |  |  |  |  |  | * | * |  |  |  |  |  | * |  |  |  | * |  | * | * | * |  | Karanja Oil |
| * |  |  |  |  |  |  |  |  |  |  |  |  |  |  |  |  |  |  |  |  | * |  |  |  | * |  |  |  |  |  | Kiwi Fruit |
|  |  |  |  |  |  |  |  | * |  |  |  |  |  |  |  |  |  |  |  |  |  |  |  |  |  |  |  |  |  |  | Lanolin |
|  |  |  |  |  | * |  | * | * |  | * |  |  |  |  |  |  |  |  |  |  | * |  |  | * | * | * |  | * |  |  | Lavender |
|  |  |  |  |  | * |  | * | * | * | * |  |  |  |  |  |  |  |  |  |  |  |  |  |  |  |  |  |  |  | * | Macadamias |
|  |  |  |  |  | * |  |  |  |  |  |  |  |  | * |  |  |  |  |  |  |  |  |  |  | * |  | * | * |  | * | Manuka Oil |
| * |  |  |  |  |  |  |  | * |  |  |  |  |  |  |  | * |  |  |  |  |  |  |  |  | * |  |  | * |  |  | Melons |
|  |  |  |  |  | * |  | * |  |  | * |  |  |  |  |  | * |  |  |  |  |  |  |  |  | * |  |  | * |  | * | Milk |
|  |  |  |  |  |  |  |  |  |  |  |  |  |  |  |  |  |  |  |  |  |  |  | * |  | * |  | * | * |  |  | Myrrh |
|  |  | * |  |  |  |  | * |  |  |  |  |  | * | * |  |  |  |  |  |  | * |  |  |  | * |  | * | * |  | * | Neem Oil |
|  |  |  |  |  |  |  |  |  |  |  |  |  |  | * |  |  |  |  |  |  |  |  |  |  | * |  |  |  |  |  | Neroli |
|  |  |  |  |  | * |  |  |  |  |  |  |  | * |  |  |  |  |  |  |  |  |  | * |  |  |  |  |  |  | * | Oatmeal |
|  |  |  |  |  | * |  | * | * |  |  |  |  |  | * |  |  |  |  |  |  | * |  |  |  | * |  | * | * |  | * | Olive Oil |
| * |  |  |  |  |  |  | * |  |  |  |  |  |  |  |  | * | * |  |  |  | * |  | * |  | * |  |  | * | * | * | Orange |
|  |  |  |  |  |  |  |  | * |  | * |  |  |  |  | * | * | * |  |  |  | * |  | * |  | * |  |  | * | * | * | Papaya/Pawpaw |
|  |  |  |  |  |  |  |  |  |  |  |  |  |  |  |  |  | * |  |  |  |  |  |  |  |  | * |  |  |  |  | Parsley |
|  |  |  |  |  | * |  |  |  |  | * |  |  |  |  |  | * | * |  |  |  | * |  | * |  | * | * |  | * |  | * | Pomegranate |
|  | * |  |  |  |  |  |  |  |  | * |  |  |  |  | * | * |  |  |  |  |  |  |  |  |  |  |  |  |  |  | Pumpkin |
|  |  |  |  |  | * |  | * | * |  |  |  |  |  | * |  |  |  |  |  |  | * |  | * | * | * |  |  | * | * | * | Rosehip Oil |
| * |  |  |  |  |  |  | * | * |  |  |  |  |  |  |  |  |  |  |  |  |  |  |  |  | * |  |  | * | * | * | Safflower oil |
|  |  |  |  |  |  |  |  |  |  |  |  |  |  |  |  | * |  |  |  |  |  | * |  |  | * |  |  |  |  | * | Strawberries |
|  |  |  |  |  |  |  | * | * |  |  |  |  |  | * |  |  |  |  |  |  |  |  |  |  | * |  |  | * | * | * | Sunflower Meal |
|  |  |  |  |  |  |  | * | * |  |  |  |  |  |  |  |  |  |  |  |  |  |  |  |  | * |  |  | * | * | * | Sunflower Oil |
|  |  |  | * |  |  |  |  |  |  |  |  |  |  |  |  |  |  |  |  |  | * | * |  | * |  |  | * |  |  | * | Tea Tree Oil |
| * |  |  |  |  | * |  |  |  |  |  |  |  |  | * |  |  | * |  |  |  | * |  | * | * |  |  |  | * |  | * | Vitamin A. |
|  |  |  |  |  | * |  | * |  |  | * |  |  |  |  |  | * |  |  |  |  |  |  |  |  |  |  |  | * |  | * | Yoghurt |

# 7. HOW TO USE INGREDIENTS: FUNDAMENTALS

Many base ingredients like mashed pumpkin, sweet potato and fruits are rich in anti-oxidants and natural fruit sugars which are also great for gently exfoliating and renewing skin cells.

## BASES

You can make a whole range of mask bases depending on what you have available and add "active" beneficial ingredients to them. For example, you can make moisturizing bases out of oil blends, coconut, milk, Yogurt or cream and then add other oils, fruits, nuts or vegetables to your base.

Some good bases include:

## MOISTURIZING BASES

Fresh cream, yogurt, fatty oils such as sunflower, safflower, macadamia, almond, flaxseed and olive.

## ANTIOXIDANT BASES

Fruits, nuts.

## REPAIRING BASES

Essential fatty oil blends such as nut oils, olive oils, seed oils, olive oil and coconut oil.

## SERUMS

You can create serums as well using oils including a base of evening primrose, rosehip, grapeseed and jojoba to add other ingredients to with anti aging, anti oxidant, and moisturizing properties.

## STORAGE TIPS

Save any leftover recipes in ice cube trays in the freezer or stored in the refrigerator for use later.  Fruits will last a few days and powders (non fruit and vegetable) will last for several months especially if stored in glass jars.

## HOUSEHOLD CLEANING

Add a few drops of Rosemary oil. Eucalyptus oil, Lavender oil and Tea tree oil t a cup of water with a squeeze of lemon juice for a fantastic grease fighting antibacterial cleaner around your home.

If using on delicate surfaces and varnish omit the Eucalyptus oil

# 9. PREPARATION TOOLS: WHAT YOU WILL NEED

There are a few items that are worth having around your home (or buying if you don't have them) to make the job of mixing and applying your products easier.

**STIRRING SPOONS AND WHISKS**

**CUTTING BOARD**

Make sure its been well cleaned before you use it to prevent the spread of bacteria

**SPATULAS**

**SMALL WHISK**

**BOWLS**

You'll need an array of small to medium bowls from glass, stainless steel and of course plastic containers for storing your finish products

**COFFEE FILTER OR SIEVE**

For straining tea and various herbal ingredients

**CHEESECLOTH, MUSLIN CLOTH OR PANTYHOSE**

**COFFEE GRINDER OR MORTAR AND PESTLE**

**EYEDROPPER (GLASS)**

Important if you want to add essential oils in the right quantities to your mixtures

**DOUBLE BOILER**

One stainless steel or heatproof glass bowl inside a saucepan is fine –

for heating beeswax and other "fancier" ingredients. When making fatty oily recipes its vital to use low heat and it prevents burning or scorching of you or your ingredients.

## BLENDER OR FOOD PROCESSOR

(Optional but useful)

## FUNNEL

For pouring into bottles

## MEASURING CUPS AND SPOONS

Obviously for measuring quantities accurately

Kitchen scales (you'll get good at adding ingredients by weight after a while and eventually not need one at all)

## MEASUREMENT GUIDELINES

NOTE: 2 Tablespoon = 1 ounce

1/3 Tablespoon = 1 Teaspoon

1 Tablespoon = 3 Teaspoons = ½ fluid ounce = 30 milliliters

2 Tablespoon = 3 Teaspoons = 60 milliliters

4 Tablespoon = ¼ cup = 120 milliliters

8 ounces = 1 cup = 250 milliliters

16 ounces = 2 cups = 1 pints = 550 milliliters

32 ounces = 4 cups = 2 pints = 1 quart = 1100 milliliters

## STORAGE CONTAINERS

There are a huge range of containers and packaging you can use for storing your products. I like to use smaller aluminum, plastic or glass containers and jars. If you are giving your products away as gifts you can buy a whole range of attractive visually appealing containers from the suppliers listed in our resources section.

You can buy bottles, canning jars, cream jars, muslin bags, plastic tubs, shaker jars, spritzing bottles (great for toners or hair), tins and decorative bottles (also known as woozys) and good old plastic bags

# 10. RECIPES: NATURAL FACE AND BODY CARE

When you think of a traditional recipe book, you think of it as a list of steps and instructions for arriving at a specific finished result – or meal.

This recipe book is a conglomeration of many recipes tried and tested formulas by many natural skin care experts and natural therapy practitioners over hundreds and even thousands of years.

I have delved into the histories and traditions of many cultures to deliver to you the best of the best in skin care regimens so you can enjoy the luxuries that Cleopatra and other beautiful icons of our past enjoyed plus many more ancient and modern concoctions.

You will note that you can use dried or fresh ingredients (although fresh ingredients always tend to offer the most ready to absorb nutrition for your skin.

I encourage you to customize these recipes to suit your unique needs. The more you make, use and adapt these recipes the easier it will get to create the mask, cleanser, moisturizer or exfoliator that's perfect for your skin and the seasons you are in.

## FACE CARE

There are several considerations to keep in mind in order to properly take care of your face, neck, chest & shoulders (the latter two areas are described throughout this book and commonly in the beauty industry as the décolletage which are often neglected in skin care routines).

Neem and Tea Tree Fungal & Itch Fighter For Skin & Hair

This is a great recipe for itching and irritated skin.

Add 10 drops of Neem oil and 10 drops of tea tree oil to 2 Tablespoon vegetable or nut oil (e.g virgin coconut, jojoba, sweet almond, safflower, sunflower or olive oil).

Apply thoroughly to your skin or scalp.  You can use this recipe to treat cuts, acne bites

# 11. RECIPES: SALAD DRESSING RECIPES

You can make your own dressings that contain beneficial oils for your skin and general health.  Consuming fatty acids in your diet helps your skin maintain healthy sebum levels while lowing your cholesterol. Most plant-based oils are low in saturated fat but there are oils such as palm and coconut oils which are high in saturated and fats and therefore should be avoided.

## Monounsaturated Fatty Acids

Olive, canola and peanut oil are high in monounsaturated fatty acids, which may lower your total and LDL cholesterol levels.

## Polyunsaturated Fatty Acids

Polyunsaturated fatty acids are known to be heart-healthy.  They contain sources of vitamin E and make a good choice for a salad dressing.  Oils high in polyunsaturated fats are:

Corn oil

Safflower oil

Sunflower oil

Soybean oils

If you are buying an oil-based salad dressing, you can check the label to ensure that it doesn't contain trans fats from partially hydrogenated oils

Flaxseed Oil

Flaxseed oil is the most concentrated source of alpha-linolenic acid, an essential omega-3 fatty acid. Other sources of omega-3 fatty acids are walnuts or oily fish, such as tuna or salmon.

## RECIPES FOR SALAD DRESSINGS

Making salad dressings and vinaigrettes are easy. You can come up with your own basic dressings using the oils above with some of the ingredients below:

Mustard

Garlic

Lime

Lemon

Balsamic vinegar

Coriander

Basil or other fresh herbs

Sugar

Paprika

Chilli

Parmesan cheese

Parsley

Pepper

Almond slithers

Sesame seeds

Apple cider vinegar (great for skin)

Tomato

Fresh cream

Yogurt

Cucumber

Mint

Egg yolks (whisk in to oil drop by drop to make a creamy dressing)

Pine nuts

Walnuts

Pumpkin seed


**BASIC OIL DRESSING BASE (add your own additives to taste)**

**The Vinaigrette Formula**

The basic ratio of oil to vinegar when making vinaigrettes is 3 to 1. All you need to remember is three parts oil to one part vinegar and you'll have a good foundation for delicious dressings.

You can add creamy ingredients or eggs to make creamy dressings with a hint of sugar to enhance or sweeten the taste.

The secret is to mix a basic formula using one of the oils above and then slowly whisk in vinegar and any other ingredients. Flavors develop over time after sitting for a while —leaving a dressing to rest in the fridge will bring out the flavor. Keep this in mind when adding herbs & spices, its easy to add too much.

You can test the flavor of your vinaigrette by dipping a piece of lettuce into your mixture, shaking off the excess and then taking a bite. Add more ingredients to taste.


**Here are some delicious recipes to get you started:**

**BASE SALAD DRESSING MIX**

¾ cup of extra virgin olive oil (or safflower oil, sunflower oil, or any of the oils above)

¼ cup of white wine vinegar

a dash of salt and pepper

Whisk together in a bowl before adding fresh ingredients and allow to sit for at least ½ an hour

**RASPBERRY VINAIGRETTE**

½ cup of raspberries - fresh or frozen

¼ cup of vegetable oil

¼ cup of apple cider vinegar

¼ cup of balsamic vinegar

2 Teaspoons of sugar

1 Teaspoon of Dijon mustard

## HERBED VINAIGRETTE SALAD DRESSING

To your standard vinaigrette base, add 1 Tablespoon Dijon mustard, 2 Tablespoon chopped parsley, ½ Teaspoon of your favorite dried herbs (such as thyme, basil, or marjoram) and whisk together well.

MUSTARD FLAVORED SALAD DRESSING (MUSTARD VINAIGRETTE)

1 Tablespoon Dijon mustard

To make Honey Dijon add 1 Tablespoon honey to the mustard vinaigrette

## ITALIAN AND ASIAN STYLED SALAD DRESSINGS

For an Italian Vinaigrette, start with the base dressing and add

½ Teaspoon minced garlic

½ Teaspoon of dried oregano and

1 Tablespoon chopped parsley

## ASIAN VINAIGRETTE DRESSING (USE RICE VINEGAR)

1 ½ Tablespoon soy sauce,

2 Tablespoon sesame oil,

½ Tablespoon Fresh minced or grated ginger,

½ clove minced garlic

A hint of chili sauce

Allow to sit for at least 30 minutes to allow the flavors to blend together.

## LIME AND OLIVE OIL DRESSING

I like to whisk this right in the salad bowl and then just put the salad on top and toss.

1 Tablespoon lime juice (from a bottle is fine)

1 Tablespoon water

2 Tablespoon extra virgin olive oil

Add lime juice and water to a bowl, then salt and pepper.  Whisk in Olive oil then add seasoning and sweetener to taste.

## RAITA (DELICIOUS DRESSING AND FACE MASK TOO)

Raita is a cold yogurt condiment that is often served with Indian food to balance the heat of the spicy dishes.

1 large unpeeled cucumber, halved, seeded, coarsely grated

2 cups plain whole-milk yogurt

¼ cup (packed) chopped fresh mint

1 Teaspoon ground cumin

¼ Teaspoon plus pinch of cayenne pepper

Wrap grated cucumber in kitchen towel and squeeze dry. Whisk yogurt, mint, cumin, and ¼ Teaspoon cayenne pepper in a bowl to blend. Add cucumbers and toss to coat.

Add salt and pepper to taste. Cover and refrigerate for at least 2 hours. Omit cayenne pepper if you are using this recipe for a face mask.


## TZATZIKI DIP/DRESSING (ALSO GOOD AS A COOLING EXFOLIATING FACE MASK)

A cool and creamy tangy cucumber dip flavored with garlic, it perfectly compliments grilled meats and vegetables. It's served on the side with warm pita bread triangles for dipping.  Goes well with souvlaki.

3 Tablespoon olive oil

1 Tablespoon vinegar

2 cloves garlic, minced finely

½ Teaspoon salt

¼ Teaspoon white pepper

1 cup greek yogurt, strained

1 cup sour cream

2 cucumbers, peeled, seeded and diced

1 Teaspoon chopped fresh dill

Combine olive oil, vinegar, garlic, salt, and pepper in a bowl until well combined. Whisk the yogurt together with the sour cream then add the olive oil mixture to the yogurt mixture and mix well. Lastly, add the cucumber and chopped fresh dill. Refrigerate for at least two hours before serving.

## NUTTY DRESSINGS

You can add ground or chopped nuts to a dressing to make it extra tasty and crunchy or finely chopped herbs.

These are just a few basic recipes to start with. You can create your own anytime you like using the beneficial oils described in this book for healthier skin and body.

# 12. FACE MASKS AND TREATMENT RECIPES

## TIPS & INSTRUCTIONS

### BASES

As a rule, general ingredients you can use as mask bases in non oil blend recipes include:

Mashed avocado, papaya, Yogurt, mashed pumpkin, apple, pureed rice, ground nuts or oatmeal.

### GRINDING OF NUTS & PULSES

When using nuts, seeds or oatmeal grind seeds or nuts ground to a fine meal with a coffee grinder, blender or mortar and pestle to use as a base which can be used on their own or as base to add mashed fruits and vegetables to. Make sure they are finely ground so they do not tear your skin when being applied or rubbed onto your face.

### HONEY

When using honey, generally honey should be runny honey or warmed to a runny consistency either in the microwave or by placing in a glass bowl that's been sitting in hot water. Where possible use UMF honey – this is a honey that has very strong antibacterial and beneficial enzymes, vitamins and other nutrients in it. UMF honey is especially good for calming repairing acneic skin as it has strong antibacterial properties.

### EXTRA VIRGIN OILS

When using coconut and olive oils try to use extra virgin oils as they contain the most potent benefits for your skin.

## EYE AREAS

The areas around your eyes are vey delicate so unless specified in recipes, avoid applying any skin care treatment to the delicate skin areas around the eye sockets and just under your eyes. You will find eye serums in this book that deal specifically with the delicate eye areas and "wrinkle zones" so please assume unless otherwise directed that you need to avoid the eye area.

## WARM WATER OR COTTON PADS

When a recipe says "rinse off with warm water" you can use your hands, cotton pads dipped in warm water, cleanser or a face cloth depending on what you prefer.

## TEAS, INFUSIONS & BREWS

Teas and infusions can be described as herbs, fruits, spices or teas that have been soaked/steeped in hot water for 10 minutes. Brews are herbs, fruits, spices or other ingredients that have been simmered on heat for a period of time.

## CUCUMBER

Use cucumber unpeeled unless directed otherwise. The skins of fruits, vegetables and nuts often contain more beneficial ingredients than their flesh so where possible use the skin.

## ALOE VERA

Aloe is best used fresh – use the fresh gel from inside a fresh aloe leaf. Aloe is easy to grow and keep on a window sill. Otherwise use store bought gel of Aloe juice from the supermarket.

## PHOTOSENSITIVITY

Certain oils & fruits (mainly fruit oils) can cause photosensitivity (sun sensitivity) and so you should limit sun exposure immediately after using these and/or apply sun protection:  These are indicated in their descriptions and uses above and include Lime, Grapefruit, Bergamot.

## SPF OILS

There are also carrier oils that provide low to medium SPF protection. Below is a table list of oils and their SPF rating:Red Raspberry Seed Oil: SPF 28-50

Carrot Seed Oil: SPF 38-40

Wheatgerm Oil: SPF 20

Soybean Oil: SPF 2-4

Olive Oil: SPF 2-8

Coconut Oil: SPF 2-8

Avocado Oil (unrefined): SPF 4-15

Castor Oil: SPF 6

Almond Oil: SPF

## SUBSTITUTES

Below is a list of alternative ingredients you can use as substitutes if you don't have the ingredient listed in the recipe. All of the ingredients separated by commas are suitable substitutes for the ingredient in the same group:

Lemon, Grapefruit, Orange, Lime

Clays, Cat Litter (a brand that contains/is made of bentonite clay – check the label) crushed into powder

Yogurt, Sour Cream, Ricotta Cheese, Milk, Cream

Oatmeal, Chickpea Flour, Ground Sunflower Meal, Ground Almonds

## APPLICATION

Apply masks with fingertips or brush in a gentle upward or outward motion. Apply cleansers and exfoliators with fingertips in a gentle circular upward motion and remove with warm water.

# INGREDIENTS FOR SPECIFIC SKIN TYPES & CONDITIONS

## ACNE

Almond meal, Aloe Vera, Apple, Apple Cider, Apricots Raw, Arrowroot, Basil, Bergamot, Cajeput, Calendula, Cedarwood, Cucumber, Eucalyptus, Evening Primrose Oil, Frankincense, German Chamomile, Gotu Kola, Grapefruit, Guava, Helichrysum, Juniper, Lavender, Lemon Myrtle, Macadamias, Manuka Oil, Milk, Mints, Niaouli, Orange, Oregano, Niaouli, Palma Rosa, Petitgrain, Pomegranate, Rose Geranium, Rosehip Oil, Rosemary, Rosewood, Sandalwood, Spike Lavender, Tea Tree, Thyme, Ylang Ylang, Vetiver, Vinegar, Vitamin A, Yarrow Hydrosol, Yogurt

## AGE SPOTS

Alpha-Lipoic Acid, Baking Soda, Carrot Seed Oil, Cucumber, Pomegranate, Rosehip Oil, Safflower Oil, Sandalwood Oil, Sesame Oil, Sunflower Meal, Sunflower Oil, Vitamin A

## ANTI-AGING & WRINKLES

Almond Meal, Almond Oil, Alpha-Hydroxy Acid, Apricot Kernel Oil, Avocado, Carrot Seed Oil, Clary Sage, Coconut, Cream, Egg Whites, Evening Primrose, Evening Primrose Oil, Figs, Frankincense, Grape Seed Oil, Honey, Jojoba Oil, Karanja Oil, Neem Oil, Olive Oil, Orange, Rosehip Oil, Safflower Oil, Sunflower Meal, Sunflower Oil, Vitamin A

## ANTI-FUNGAL

Almond Meal, Almond Oil, Anti-inflammatory, Calendula, Calophyllum (Tamanu) Oil, Cream, Honey, Karanja Oil, Lavender, Manuka Oil, Milk,

Myrhh, Neem Oil, Neroli, Pomegranate, Rosehip Oil, Tea Tree Oil, Yogurt

## ANTI-OXIDANT

Almond Meal, Alpha-Hydroxy Acid, Alpha-Lipoic Acid, Apple, Apple Cider Vinegar, Apricots Raw, Argan Oil, Aubergine, Avocado, Carrot Seed Oil, Chamomile, Elder Flower, Figs, Guava, Honey, Kiwi Fruit, Melons, Orange, Pomegranate, Rosehip Oil, Safflower Oil, Sunflower Meal, Sunflower Oil

## ANTI-SEPTIC/ANTI-BACTERIAL

Avocado, Bergamot, Blackberry, Carrot Seed Oil, Coconut Oil, Karanja Oil, Lavender, Manuka Oil, Myrhh, Neem Oil, Parsley, Rosemary, Tea Tree Oil, Thyme

## ASTRINGENT

Grapefruit, Lime Distilled, Rosemary, Yarrow

## BALANCING

Almond Oil, Aloe Vera, Apple Cider Vinegar, Apricot Kernel Oil, Carrot Seed Oil, Coconut, Cucumber, Elder Flower, Evening Primrose Oil, Geranium, Juniper, Lavender, Oatmeal, Pomegranate, Rosehip Oil, Vitamin A

## CELLULITE

Almond Oil, Carrot Seed Oil, Coconut Oil, Evening Primrose Oil, Juniper, Lavender, Rosehip Oil, Vitamin A

## CHAPPED/ CRACKED SKIN

Cajeput, Calendula Infused Oil, Lavender, Myrrh, Patchouli, Roman and German Chamomile, Sandalwood, Vetiver

## CHILBLAINS

Black Pepper, Cinnamon Leaf, Clove Bud, Ginger, Lavender

## CLEANSING

Almond Oil, Alpha-Hydroxy Acid, Alpha-Lipoic Acid, Apple Cider Vinegar, Apple, Apricot Kernel Oil, Apricots Raw, Banana, Basil, Bergamot, Blackberry, Brown Sugar, Coconut, Egg Whites, Elder Flower, Fennel, Grape Seed Oil, Guava, Honey, Jojoba Oil, Juniper, Lemon, Lemongrass, Niaouli, Peppermint, Sweet Basil Lavender, Melons, Olive Oil, Orange, Pomegranate, Rosehip Oil

## COMBINATION SKIN

Geranium, Neroli Hydrosol, Rose Geranium Hydrosol, Rosewood, Ylang-ylang

## COOLING (SUNBURNT, WINDBURNT OR ENVIRONMENTALLY DAMAGED SKIN)

Aloe Vera, Coconut Oil, Cucumber, Peppermint Oil, Vitamin C

## DARK CIRCLES/PUFFINESS

Coffee, Cucumber, Soya Bean Oil, Vitamin K

## DEVITALIZED SKIN

Eucalyptus Globulous, Myrtle, Neroli, Basil, Juniper, Lemon, Lemongrass, Niaouli, Peppermint, Pine, Orange, Oregano, Rosemary, Spearmint, Geranium, Grapefruit

## DISCOLORATION

Carrot Seed Oil, Cream, Cucumber, Orange, Pomegranate, Rosehip Oil, Vitamin A

## DRY ACNE

Clary Sage, Lavender, Petitgrain, Rose Geranium, Spike Lavender

## DRY SKIN

Calendula Infused Oil, Carrot Seed Oil, Carrot Seed Oil, Cedarwood, Clary Sage, Geranium, Jasmine, Lavender, Lavender, Mandarine, Petitgrain, Neroli, Orange, Palma Rosa, Petitgrain, Roman Chamomile, Rose, Rose Or Neroli Hydrosol, Rosewood, Sandalwood, Vetiver, Ylang ylang

## ECZEMA

Cedarwood, Bergamot, Carrot Seed Oil, German Chamomile, Helichrysum, Juniper, Karanja, Lavender, Myrrh, Neem, Palma Rosa,

Patchouli, Roman Chamomile, Sandalwood, Tea Tree, Yarrow, Ylang ylang

## EXFOLIATING

Almond Meal, Alpha-Hydroxy Acid, Alpha-Lipoic Acid, Apple Cider Vinegar, Apple, Apricots Raw, Banana, Brown Sugar, Cream, Demerara Sugar, Figs, Ground Oatmeal, Ground Seeds & Nuts, Guava, Honey, Jojoba Beads, Kiwi Fruit, Melons, Milk Powder, Milk, Molasses, Orange, Papaya, Paw Paw, Pineapple, Pomegranate, Salt, Sunflower Meal, Yogurt

## HEALING/SCARRING & STRETCH MARKS

Apricot Kernel Oil, Calendula, Calophyllum (Tamanu) Oil, Carrot Seed Oil, Chamomile, Geranium, Honey, Neroli, Olive Oil, Rosehip Oil, Vitamin A, Galbanum, Helichrysum (in a Base Of Rose Hip Seed Oil), Lavender, Petitgrain

## HYDRATING:

Mandarine, Most Hydrosols Especially Rose And Neroli, Palma Rosa, Rose, Sweet Orange, Tangerine

## INFECTIONS

Calendula, Eucalyptus, German Chamomile, Laurel, Lavender, Manuka, Myrrh, Myrtle, Niaouli, Palma Rosa, Roman Chamomile, Rosemary, Rosewood, Spikenard, Tea Tree, Thyme, Ylang ylang

## INFLAMED SKIN (AGGRAVATED OR ACNEIC SKIN)

Aloe Vera, Argan Oil, Calendula, Chamomile, Coconut Oil, Elder Flower, Honey, Jojoba Oil, Karanja Oil, Lavender, Neem Oil, Sea Buckthorn Oil

## INFLAMMATION

Angelica, Carrot Seed Oil, Cistus, Clary Sage, Galbanum, German and Roman Chamomile, Helichrysum, Myrrh, Myrtle, Rosewood, St. Johns Wort Infusion, Witch Hazel Or Chamomile Hydrosols, Yarrow

## INSECT REPELLANT

Cedarwood, Cream, Eucalyptus, Geranium Oil, Karanja Oil, Neem Oil, Tea Tree Oil

## ITCHY SKIN

Aloe Vera Juice Or Gel, Apple Cider Vinegar, Apricot Kernel Oil, Babassu Oil, Baking Soda, Chamomile, Emu Oil, Helichrysum, Jasmine, Karanja Oil, Lavender Or Witch Hazel Hydrosol, Neem, Peppermint, Roman Chamomile, Lavender Oil, Manuka Oil, Neem Oil, Oatmeal

## LARGE PORES

Cedarwood, Lemongrass, Myrtle, Rose

## LIGHTENING/BRIGHTENING

Almond Meal, Alpha-Hydroxy Acid, Apricots Raw, Blackberry, Chamomile, Cucumber, Egg Whites, Japanese Soya Sauce, Lemon, Milk,

Pomegranate, Rosehip Oil, Yogurt

## MAKE UP REMOVAL

Alpha-Hydroxy Acid, Cream, Oil Blends (most oils)

## MATURE AGED SKIN, LINES & WRINKLES

Carrot Seed Oil, Cistus, Clary Sage, Creme Cleanser, Cypress, Elemi, Fennel, Frankincense, Galbanum, Geranium, Lavender, Myrrh, Neroli, Patchouli, Rose, Rosehip Oil, Rosewood, Sage, Sea Buckthorn Berry Extract.

## MATURE SKIN

Almond Meal, Almond Oil, Alpha-Hydroxy Acid, Alpha-Lipoic Acid, Apple Cider Vinegar, Argan Oil, Avocado, Blackberry, Carrot Seed Oil, Clary Sage, Cocoa Butter, Coconut, Evening Primrose Oil, Frankincense, Honey, Lanolin, Macadamias, Olive Oil, Rose Oil, Rosehip Oil, Safflower Oil, Sunflower Meal, Vitamin A

## MOISTURIZING

Almond Meal, Almond Oil, Aloe Vera, Alpha-Lipoic Acid, Apple, Apricot Kernel Oil, Argan Oil, Avocado, Blackberry, Brown Sugar, Carrot Seed Oil, Castor Oil, Chocolate, Clary Sage, Cocoa Butter, Coconut, Evening Primrose Oil, Fennel, Frankincense, Grape Seed Oil, Hazelnuts, Honey, Jojoba Oil, Juniper, Karanja Oil, Lanolin, Macadamias, Mango Butter, Milk, Neem Oil, Olive Oil, Rose Oil, Rosehip Oil, Safflower Oil, Shea Butter, Soya Bean Oil, Sunflower Meal, Sunflower Oil, Yogurt

## NORMAL SKIN

All Hydrosols, Angelica, Cedarwood, Geranium, Jasmine, Lavender, Neroli, Roman Chamomile, Rose, Rosewood, Ylang ylang

## OILY SKIN/BLACKHEADS

Apple Cider Vinegar, Arrowroot, Coconut Oil, Coriander, Coriander, Vulgaris, Peppermint, Lemongrass, Cream, Egg Whites, Evening Primrose Oil, Gotu Kola, Lemongrass, Macadamias, Peppermint, Thyme

## OILY SKIN

Cedarwood, Cajeput, Calendula Infusion, Cedarwood, Clary Sage, Coriander, Cypress, Frankincense, Geranium, Grapefruit, Juniper, Lavandin, Lavender, Lemon, Lime Distilled, Melissa, Niaouli, Patchouli, Peppermint, Petitgrain, Roman and German Chamomile, Rose, Sandalwood, Spike Lavender, Texas) Geranium, Thyme, Yarrow, Ylang-ylang

## PSORIASIS

Bergamot, Cajeput, Calendula Infused Oil, Carrot Seed Oil, Cranberry Seed Oil, German Or Roman Chamomile, Helichrysum, Juniper, Lavender, Neem, Pomegranate, Sandalwood, Tea Tree

## RED VEINS, BROKEN OR CONGESTED CAPILLARIES

Borage Oil, Calendula Infused Oil, Carrot Seed Oil, Cypress, Geranium, Helichrysum, Helichrysum Or Neroli Hydrosols, Lavender, Lemon, Neroli, Parsley, Roman and German Chamomile, Rose

## REDUCING PUFFINESS

Celery, Clary Sage, Cypress, Fennel, Oregano, Peppermint, Roman Chamomile, Rosemary, Spanish Marjoram

## REPAIRING

Aloe Vera, Alpha-Hydroxy Acid, Alpha-Lipoic Acid, Avocado, Calendula, Calophyllum (Tamanu) Oil, Evening Primrose Oil, Geranium, Honey, Manuka Oil, Olive Oil, Pomegranate, Rosehip Oil, Vitamin A

## REVITALIZING SKIN

Calendula, Carrot Seed Oil, Niaouli, Orange, Rosewood, Tea Tree

## ROSACEA

German Chamomile, Helichrysum Hydrosol, Helichrysum Italicuum, Rosewood

## Sensitive Skin

Angelica, Carrot, Chamomile Or Yarrow Hydrosols, Helichrysum, Jasmine, Neroli, Neroli, Palma Rosa, Rose, Rosewood, Chamomile, Oatmeal, Aloe Vera

## SKIN REGENERATION

Calendula, Caraway, Carrot Seed Oil, Cistus, Clary Sage, Elemi,

Galbanum, Helichrysum, Lavender, Lavender, Myrrh, Myrtle, Neroli, Palma Rosa, Patchouli, Rose, Rosemary, Sandalwood, Sage, Spikenard, Tea Tree, Vetiver, Frankincense

## SKIN TONER

Chamomile, Frankincense, Hydrosols, Lavender, Lemon, Lemongrass, Neroli, Orange, Petitgrain, Rose, Calendula, Witch Hazel, Aloe Vera Juice, Apple Cider Vinegar

## SKINCARE GENERAL

Chamomile, Cypress, Geranium, Geranium Essential Oils And Hydrosols, Lavender, Rose, Rosemary Camphor, Rosewood

## SOOTHING (IRRITATED SKIN)

Almond Meal, Almond Oil, Apple Cider Vinegar, Calendula, Calophyllum (Tamanu) Oil, Chamomile, Chocolate, Lavender, Macadamias, Milk, Oatmeal, Yogurt

## SPF (LOW PROTECTION)

Coconut Oil, Neem Oil, Sesame Oil

## STIMULATING (CIRCULATION OR COLLAGEN PRODUCTION)

Alpha-Hydroxy Acid, Anise Seed Oil, Apple, Banana, Cream, Cucumber, Egg Whites, Eucalyptus, Figs, Ginger, Kiwi Fruit, Melons, Orange

# RECIPES

## ACNE APPLE CIDER VINEGAR FOR PIMPLES

Acne, Anti-oxidant, Cleansing, Exfoliating, Moisturizing, Tightening

Apply straight apple cider vinegar carefully with a Q-tip to each pimple once or twice daily. This helps to quickly dry pimples, prevent spreading, calm inflammation and redness.

## ACNE APPLE MASK

Acne, Anti-aging, Age Spots, Anti-oxidant, Anti-fungal, Antiseptic, Antibacterial, Balancing, Cellulite, Calming, Cleansing, Exfoliating, Itchy Skin Moisturizing, Soothing, Tightening

2 Tablespoons mashed Apple or pear

1 Teaspoon crushed rosemary, sage or Lavender leaves

Pinch of salt or Baking Soda

Mash together well (cooked or raw is fine) then apply to your skin. Leave on for 10 minutes then rinse off.

## ACNE APPLE SOOTHING MASK

Acne, Age Spots, Anti-fungal, Anti-oxidant, Balancing, Brightening, Cleansing, Cooling, Dark Circles, Discoloration, Exfoliating, Itchy Skin, Lightening, Moisturizing, Puffiness, Soothing, Tightening

½ cup oatmeal finely ground

½ a ripe Apple

3 Tablespoons crushed Cucumber

2 Tablespoons Milk

Mix the ingredients together in a blender and apply to skin.  Leave on for 20 minutes then wash off with warm water.


**ACNE ASPIRIN MASK**

Anti-aging, Anti-inflammatory, Anti-oxidant, Balancing, Calming, Cleansing, Exfoliating, Healing, Mature Skin, Moisturizing, Repairing, Scarring


1-3 aspirin

⅓ cup warmed honey

3 Tablespoons almond, olive or coconut oil

Crush aspirin and add to oil and honey.  Apply to skin and leave on for 10-15 minutes then rinse off.

**ACNE BAKING SODA AND TOOTHPASTE SPOT CREAM**

Age Spots, Anti-aging, Anti-inflammatory, Discoloration, Itchy Skin


1 Teaspoon of baking soda

2 Tablespoons water

½ Teaspoon toothpaste

Mix ingredients together to form a paste and dab on spots.  Clears up pimples quickly.

## ACNE BASIL BLEMISH TREATMENT

Acne, Anti-oxidant, Cleansing

1 cup water

¼ c basil

1 Tablespoon crushed mint leaves

¼ watercress crushed

3 medium size carrots (peeled and chopped)

1 egg white

Simmer all ingredients except egg white for 20 minutes on low heat. Remove from heat and allow to cool. Blend all ingredients with the egg white on medium speed for 45 seconds.

Apply to face. Let sit for 10 to 20 minutes. Rinse off with warm water.

## ACNE CLAY MASK

Acne Anti-aging, Anti-fungal, Anti-inflammatory, Anti-oxidant, Brightening, Calming, Cleansing, Exfoliating, Healing, Lightening, Mature Skin, Moisturizing, Repairing, Scarring, Soothing

3 Teaspoons green clay (if skin is sensitive, use french green clay)

1 Teaspoon honey

2 Tablespoons water (oily skin), half and half (combination skin) or Jojoba oil (dry skin)

As a general rule use 2 parts liquid to 1 part clay.

Use the liquid to suit based on your skin type.  If you have oily skin use water. Combination skin milk or half and half and for dry skin use jojoba oil.

Mix the ingredients together and apply to skin. Leave on for 10-20 minutes then rinse off with luke warm water.

## COCONUT OIL CLEANSER (WITH OPTIONAL ACNE FIGHTING INGREDIENTS)

Anti-bacterial, Anti-fungal, Cleansing, Healing, Moisturizing, Scarring

1 Teaspoon lemon juice, aloe vera juice or apple cider vinegar (omit if you have very dry skin)

2 Tablespoons extra virgin coconut oil

1 Tablespoon yogurt

For acne affected skin add a few drops of tea tree oil, lavender oil or a pinch of turmeric (can add all three)

Blend these ingredients together well and apply to skin in a circular motion. Leave on for ten minutes then wash off with water. This face wash will leave your skin feeling soft and clean.

## ACNE EAU DE COLOGNE AND LEMON JUICE

Mix equal quantities of eau de cologne and lemon juice. Apply this solution on the pimples with a Q-tip and leave it to dry reapplying a new layer every five minutes. Wash off after 15-20 minutes.

## ACNE EGG WHITE AND LEMON MASK

Anti-oxidant, Anti-aging, Cleansing, Discoloration, Exfoliating, Lightening, Oily Skin, Tightening

1 egg white

4 drops of lemon juice or essential oil

Separate the egg white from the yolk. Beat the egg white until it forms into soft peaks. Apply to skin and rinse off with warm water.


## ACNE FACE TONER RECIPE

Anti-septic, Anti-fungal, Antibacterial, Balancing, Toning


4 oz witch hazel

10 drops tea tree oil

Mix ingredients well in bottle. Shake before each use and apply to skin with cotton ball after cleansing.


## ACNE FRUIT HERBAL MASK

Anti-fungal, Anti-aging, Anti-oxidant, Anti-inflammatory, Antiseptic, Brightening, Cleansing, Discoloration, Exfoliating, Insect Repellant, Lightening ,Mature Skin, Moisturizing, Soothing, Soothing, Tightening, Wrinkles


1 Teaspoon lemon, orange, or grapefruit juice

Couple of crushed basil leaves

1 Tablespoon cream, Yogurt, milk

1 avocado

1 Tablespoon ground almond meal

Blend together to a fine mash with a blender or mortar and pestle. Apply to skin and leave on for 10 to 15 minutes then rinse off.

*Optional extras: 2 drops tea tree oil, manuka oil, rosemary oil or lavender oil

*Alternative base: use mashed apple, papaya, or pineapple.

## ACNE GREEN CLAY MASK

Anti-aging, Balancing, Cleansing, Healing, Itchy Skin, Moisturizing, Scarring, Wrinkles

1 Tablespoon green clay from any health store

1 Teaspoon apricot kernel oil

3 drops of palma rosa essential oil

Mix the ingredients together and apply to skin. Leave on for 10-20 minutes then rinse off with luke warm water.

## ACNE HERBAL FACE LOTION

Moisturizing, Anti-inflammatory, Antiseptic, Antibacterial, Exfoliating

1 oz beeswax

4 oz hazelnuts or 1 Tablespoon hazelnut oil

15 drops tea tree oil

15 drops myrhh

Melt wax and oil together on warm not hot heat (use a double boiler if you have one), when melted blend thoroughly and allow to cool to a luke warm temperature then add essential oils. Allow to cool completely and store in a glass jar.

## ACNE HONEY AND YOGURT MOISTURIZING ACNE MASK

Anti-aging, Anti-fungal, Anti-inflammatory, Anti-oxidant, Calming, Cleansing, Exfoliating, Healing, Mature Skin, Moisturizing, Repairing, Scarring, Soothing

1 Teaspoon of warmed honey

1 Teaspoon of plain Yogurt

Mix the ingredients together and apply to skin. Leave on for 10-20 minutes then rinse off with luke warm water.

## ACNE HONEY PIMPLE REMEDY (HEALING AND MOISTURIZING)

Anti-aging, Anti-inflammatory, Anti-oxidant, Calming, Cleansing, Exfoliating, Healing, Scarring, Mature Skin, Moisturizing, Repairing

3 Tablespoons honey

1 Teaspoon cinnamon

Mix the ingredients together and apply to infected areas or spots. Can be washed off after 20 minutes if you wish.

## ACNE JUICE MASK

Anti-aging, Anti-inflammatory, Anti-oxidant, Blackheads, Brightening, Calming, Cleansing, Exfoliating, Healing, Lightening, Mature Skin, Moisturizing, Oily Skin, Repairing, Scarring, Tightening, Wrinkles

1 Teaspoon lemon juice

2 egg whites

3 Teaspoons honey

1 cup strawberries

Mash & mix the ingredients together and apply to skin. Leave on for 10 minutes then rinse off with luke warm water.

## ACNE MILK OF MAGNESIA

Acne, Anti-fungal, Exfoliating, Lightening, Brightening, Moisturizing, Soothing

1 bottle Milk of Magnesia applied with a cotton ball or pad. Leave on for 10-20 minutes and rinse off.

## ACNE MILK SOOTHING MASK

Acne, Anti-aging, Anti-fungal, Anti-inflammatory, Anti-oxidant, Balancing, Brightening, Calming, Cleansing, Cooling, Exfoliating, Healing, Lightening, Mature Skin, Moisturizing, Repairing, Scarring, Soothing

1 Teaspoon powdered milk

1 Tablespoon runny honey

1 Teaspoon aloe vera

2 drops essential oil of your choice

Mix the ingredients together and apply to skin. Leave on for 10-20 minutes then rinse off with luke warm water.

## ACNE NUTMEG PIMPLE REMEDY

Acne, Anti-fungal, Brightening, Exfoliating, Lightening, Moisturizing, Soothing

1 Tablespoon ground nutmeg

1 Tablespoon milk

Mix the ingredients together and apply to infected areas or spots. Can be washed off after 20 minutes if you wish.

## ACNE OATMEAL MASK

Anti-aging, Anti-inflammatory, Balancing, Cellulite, Cleansing, Itchy Skin, Mature Skin, Moisturizing, Soothing

5 five drops of almond oil

Juice of half a lemon

1 egg white

1 Tablespoon oatmeal powder (ground oatmeal)

Mix all the ingredients in a bowl to make a smooth paste. Add water if it is very thick. Apply it on the face and leave on for 15–20 minutes. Rinse off with luke warm water.

## ACNE OIL BLEND

Acne, Anti-aging, Anti-fungal, Anti-inflammatory, Antibacterial, Antiseptic, Balancing, Calming, Cellulite, Cleansing, Healing, Itchy Skin, Mature Skin, Moisturizing, Repairing, Scarring

2 Tablespoons jojoba oil or coconut oil (or use grapeseed or any other

oil mentioned in this book as a base oil)

6 drops lavender oil

5 drops tea tree (melaleuca) or manuka oil

1 drop geranium oil (optional)

Blend ingredients together gently and apply to problem areas of the skin or add to a mask.  Store in a glass container.


## ACNE PATCHOULI HERBAL CLEANSER

Anti-oxidant, Exfoliating, Healing, Moisturizing, Renewing, Rejuvenating, Repairing


2 Tablespoons ground hazelnuts or 1 Tablespoon hazelnut Oil

2 Tablespoons grapeseed oil

5 drops Myrrh essential oil

5 drops patchouli

5 Drops tea tree oil

Mix ingredients well in bottle.  Shake before each use then apply to skin in a circular motion for a minute or two.  Rinse off with warm water.


## ACNE SERUM MOISTURIZER

Anti-aging, Anti-fungal, Antiseptic, Antibacterial, Balancing, Calming, Cleansing, Healing, Scarring, Itchy Skin, Moisturizing, Repairing, Soothing, Wrinkles


1 oz apricot kernel oil

12 drops lavender oil

7 drops tea tree oil

1 drop geranium oil

Mix all ingredients in a clear plastic or glass bottle shaking well for 2 minutes then apply 1-2 drops after washing.

## ACNE SLIPPERY ELM MASK

Acne, Moisturizing, Oily Skin

1 oz slippery elm powder

3 oz water

3 drops tea tree oil (optional) can also use crushed rosemary leaves

Mix ingredients together and apply to skin. Leave on for 10 mins then wash off with warm water.

## ACNE STRAWBERRY CLEANSER

Acne, Anti-fungal, Brightening, Exfoliating, Lightening, Moisturizing, Soothing

2 Tablespoons strawberry Yogurt or

1 strawberry and 1 Tablespoon plain Yogurt

Mix the ingredients together and apply to skin in a circular motion for 2 minutes. Rinse off with luke warm water.

## ACNE STRAWBERRY MASK

Anti-aging, Anti-inflammatory, Insect Repellant, Discoloration, Moisturizing

¼ cup strawberries

¼ cup sour cream or plain yogurt

Mash the strawberries and yogurt or sour cream together. Apply to face and wash off after 10-15 minutes.

## ACNE TEA TREE OIL FOR PIMPLES

Anti-fungal, Antiseptic, Antibacterial, Balancing, Calming Cellulite, Cleansing, Soothing

15 drops tea tree oil

5 drops lavender oil

5 drops water

Blend ingredients together. Apply to each pimple a few times a day with a q-tip to quickly dry out spots.

## ACNE TOMATO FACE MASK

Acne, Anti-fungal, Balancing, Brightening, Cooling, Calming, Dark Circles, Discoloration, Exfoliating, Itchy Skin, Lightening, Moisturizing, Puffiness, Oily Skin, Repairing, Tightening

1 mashed tomato with seeds removed

2 Teaspoons plain Yogurt

1 Teaspoon mashed Cucumber

1 Teaspoon aloe vera gel

2 Teaspoons oatmeal

2 crushed mint leaves

Mix the ingredients together and apply to skin. Leave on for 10 minutes and wash off. Also great for oily skin.

## ACNE TURMERIC AND HONEY MASK

Acne, Anti-aging, Anti-fungal, Anti-inflammatory, Anti-oxidant, Brightening, Calming, Cleansing, Exfoliating, Healing, Lightening, Mature Skin, Moisturizing, Repairing, Scarring, Soothing

1 Teaspoon of natural (not powdered) Milk

1 Teaspoon of honey

1 Teaspoon of turmeric

Mix the ingredients together and apply to skin. Leave on for 10-20 minutes then rinse off with luke warm water.

## ACNE REJUVENATING REPAIRING SEAWEED MASK

Acne, Balancing, Blackheads, Calming, Cooling, Moisturizing, Repairing

4 Tablespoons kelp powder

½ cup of aloe vera gel or juice

3 Tablespoons distilled water

Combine dry ingredients adding water gradually until the mixture has a consistency of a thick paste.

Apply on the face and neck and leave it on for about 15 minutes. Rinse off with warm water.

## ACNE CALMING OILY SKIN MASK

Acne, Balancing, Cooling, Calming, Moisturizing, Repairing

½ cup aloe vera gel

1 ½ Tablespoon cornstarch

1 Tablespoon witch hazel

3-4 drops peppermint oil

Mix aloe, cornstarch and witch hazel in glass bowl. Microwave in 3 to 4 30 second intervals stirring every interval or cook in a double boiler stirring constantly until it forms a light paste. Store in refrigerator and apply as needed then rinse off with water.

## ACV PH BALANCER

Acne, Anti-oxidant, Cleansing, Exfoliating, Moisturizing, Tightening

3 cups distilled water

⅓ cup Apple cider vinegar

Combine water and cider vinegar. Pour into a clean container.  Moisten a cotton ball and use after cleansing to restore your skin's ph balance.

## AGE SPOT MASK

Acne, Age Spots, Anti-aging, Anti-inflammatory, Anti-oxidant, Balancing, Brightening, Cleansing, Cooling, Dark Circles, Discoloration, Exfoliating, Lightening, Moisturizing, Puffiness, Repairing, Tightening,

1 Teaspoon cucumber

Half a mashed or pureed carrot

1 Tablespoon sunflower oil

Half an apple or 1 Teaspoon of pineapple or 1 Tablespoon papaya or pomegranate

Mash ingredients together and apply as a mask for approx. 10 to 15 minutes. Rinse off.

## AGE SPOT OR SUN SPOT SERUM & DISCOLORATION

Acne, Age Spots, Anti-aging, Balancing, Brightening, Cleansing, Cooling, Dark Circles, Discoloration, Lightening, Moisturizing, Puffiness, Tightening

2 Tablespoons jojoba oil

Add 5 drops citrus juice (preferably lemon)

½ Teaspoon cucumber juice (squeezed from Cucumber pulp)

4 drops sesame oil

3 drops sandalwood oil

Blend all ingredients together and apply to age spots daily for a gentle but effective lightener. Also good for freckles, other spots and for general skin whitening. Store in refrigerator.

## AGE SPOT SANDALWOOD, LEMON, CARROT SEED OIL & CUCUMBER BLEND

Acne, Age Spots, Anti-aging, Anti-oxidant, Antibacterial, Antiseptic, Balancing, Brightening, Cellulite, Cooling, Dark Circles, Discoloration, Healing, Lightening, Mature Skin, Moisturizing, Puffiness, Scarring, Tightening, Wrinkles

4 drops sandalwood oil

6 drops carrot seed oil

4 drops lemon oil or 10 drops of lemon juice

½ cup squeezed cucumber juice

Mix, shake well and apply to effected areas once or twice a day.


## AGE SPOT OILS

Use any of the following straight (dab directly on skin):


Aloe Vera juice

Castor oil

Apple juice

Apple cider vinegar

Buttermilk

Lemon juice

Equal parts apple and onion juice

Dab a cotton pad into the solution and apply directly onto age spots.

Repeat this once a day for approximately 6 weeks and you should begin to notice a gradual improvement. If the spots have not completely disappeared after the 6 weeks keep using the solution until they have.

Dandelion tea

Gotu kola

Horseradish

## ANTI AGING PEACH FACE MASK

Anti-aging, Anti-inflammatory, Discoloration

2 mid sized peaches mashed

2 Tablespoons whipped cream

Mix the ingredients together, apply to skin. Leave on for 10 minutes then rinse off with warm water.

## ANTI-AGING ANTI-OXIDANT EGG WHITE, RED WINE FACE MASK

Anti-aging, Anti-inflammatory, Anti-oxidant, Calming, Cleansing, Exfoliating, Healing, Mature Skin, Moisturizing, Scarring, Tightening

1 egg white

3 Tablespoons red wine

1 Tablespoon organic honey

Gently mix the egg white, red wine and Honey together until you have a smooth paste.

Spread the paste gently and equally with your fingertips on your clean face and neck avoiding the eye area clear

Leave the mask on for 10-15 minutes then wash off with warm water.

## ANTI-AGING CARROT FACE MASK

Anti-aging, Cleansing, Discoloration, Healing, Mature Skin, Moisturizing, Repairing, Scarring

½ cup carrot juice

1 egg yolk

½ Tablespoon olive oil

Mix it all and apply to face and neck. Rinse off after 20-25min using luke warm water.

## ANTI-AGING CHINESE ROYAL YOUTH TONIC

Anti-aging, Anti-inflammatory, Anti-oxidant, Calming, Cleansing, Discoloration, Exfoliating, Healing, Lightening, Mature Skin, Moisturizing, Repairing, Scarring, Wrinkles

3 eggs

1 Tablespoon honey

1 cup red wine

Break eggs into a bowl with an airtight cover. Fill and cover the eggs with the red wine and leave in the refrigerator for 4 or 5 days then add honey. Mix well and apply to skin daily. Store for up to a month in refrigerator.

## ANTI-AGING CREAMY FACE MASK RECIPE

Anti-aging, Anti-inflammatory, Cleansing, Discoloration, Exfoliating, Moisturizing, Tightening

¼ cup heavy whipping cream

1 med banana peeled

1 vitamin E capsule

Mash together cream and banana then mix in vitamin E capsule. Apply to face and neck. Leave on for 10 to 15 minutes. Rinse off with warm water.

## ANTI-AGING EGG YOLK BUTTERMILK SOAK

Anti-aging, Blackheads, Brightening, Cleansing, Lightening, Oily Skin, Tightening, Wrinkles

2 egg yolks

3 Tablespoons Buttermilk

Mix well until light and fluffy and dab on face with a cotton pad or ball. Rinse off with warm water.

## ANTI-AGING GLYCERIN CREAM MASK

Anti-aging, Anti-inflammatory, Anti-oxidant, Calming, Cleansing, Discoloration, Exfoliating, Healing, Insect Repellant, Mature Skin, Moisturizing, Repairing, Scarring

1 oz of glycerin

3 Tablespoons honey

3 Tablespoons wheat germ oil or olive oil or almond oil

1 oz witch hazel or 5 drops lemon juice

½ oz of rose water

Blend well and apply around eyes and mouth (wrinkle zones) daily.

## ANTI-AGING MATURE SKIN HONEY FRUIT AGE DEFYING MASK

Acne, Anti-aging, Anti-inflammatory, Anti-oxidant, Calming, Cleansing, Discoloration, Exfoliating, Healing, Mature Skin, Moisturizing, Repairing, Scarring, Tightening

1 Teaspoon of honey

A few drops of orange juice

Blend well and apply to skin, leave on for at least 10 minutes and up to an hour then rinse off with warm water.

## ANTI-AGING MILK, SANDALWOOD AND TURMERIC MASK

Acne, Anti-aging, Anti-fungal, Anti-inflammatory, Brightening, Cooling, Discoloration, Exfoliating, Insect Repellant, Lightening, Moisturizing, Soothing

½ cup full fat milk

½ Teaspoon turmeric powder

5 drops sandalwood oil

Boil the Milk simmer for about ten minutes in a pot on low heat and let it cool.  Skim the "cream" off the top and apply to skin.

## ANTI-AGING MOISTURIZING CREAM CHEESE AND CARROT FACE MASK

Anti-aging, Anti-inflammatory, Discoloration, Insect Repellant

1 medium size cooked mashed carrot

2 Tablespoons cream cheese

Mix the ingredients together and apply to skin.  Leave on for 10-20 minutes then rinse off with luke warm water.

## ANTI-AGING MYRRH MASK FOR AGING SKIN

Anti-aging, Anti-inflammatory, Anti-oxidant, Calming, Cleansing, Exfoliating, Healing, Mature Skin, Moisturizing, Repairing, Scarring

½ cups yogurt

2 drops of vitamin E

2 Tablespoons honey

2-3 drops Myrrh oil

Mix the ingredients together and apply to skin. Leave on for 10 minutes and wash off. Also great for oily and infected skin.

## ANTI-AGING OIL

Anti-aging, Anti-oxidant, Discoloration, Healing, Mature Skins, Moisturizing, Red Veins, Rejuvenating, Renewing, Scarring, Soothing, Stimulating, Wrinkles

1 drop of rosemary essential oil

3 drops of sandalwood essential oil

2 drops of rosemary essential oil

2 drops of rose essential oil

1 oz of rose hip oil.

Mix all the oils and blend them with rose hip oil. Apply it liberally and wash off with lukewarm water. You can also add this mixture to any face mask in this book as a moisturizing boost.

## ANTI-AGING OIL BLEND 2

Anti-aging, Anti-oxidant, Discoloration, Healing, Mature Skins, Moisturizing, Red Veins, Rejuvenating, Renewing Rejuvenating, Renewing, Scarring, Soothing, Stimulating, Wrinkles

This a fabulous anti-aging wrinkle, scar and red vein reducing serum. Great as a night treatment for skin.

1 oz rose hip oil

1 oz argan oil

3 drops carrot seed oil

2 drops frankincense oil

2 drops Myrrh oil

2 drops neroli oil

1 drop patchouli oil

3 drops rose oil

2 drops sandalwood oil

Mix and store in a dark glass bottle. Keep in a cool, dark place. Shake before using and apply to skin as an after cleansing serum. Very nourishing and moisturizing.

## ANTI-AGING PEANUT COQ10 MASK

Anti-aging, Anti-inflammatory, Anti-oxidant, Calming, Cleansing, Exfoliating, Healing, Mature Skin, Moisturizing, Repairing, Scarring

2 Tablespoon peanut oil

1 egg yolk

½ Tablespoon honey

Few drops of lemon juice

Mix peanut oil and egg yolk followed by other ingredients. Leave for 10 minutes then apply to skin and leave on for 10 minutes. Wash off with warm water.

## ANTI-AGING SWEET MANGO MASK

Anti-aging, Anti-inflammatory, Anti-oxidant, Calming, Cleansing, Exfoliating, Healing, Mature Skin, Moisturizing, Repairing, Scarring

1 small sweet potato

1 mango mashed

5 Tablespoons honey

Mash, blend or puree all ingredients together and apply to skin. Leave on for 15 minutes and wash off with warm water.

## ANTI-FUNGAL ANTISEPTIC SKIN BLEND

Acne, Anti-aging Anti-fungal, Antiseptic, Antibacterial, Calming, Healing, Moisturizing, Soothing

7 drops tea tree oil

4 drops lavender Oil

8 drops neem oil or karanja oil

20 drops olive oil or almond, or apricot oil

Blend the oils together and apply to affected areas twice daily with a cotton pad or q-tip.

## ANTI-FUNGAL SOOTHING SKIN REMEDY

Acne, Anti-aging, Anti-fungal, Anti-inflammatory, Antibacterial, Antiseptic, Balancing, Brightening, Calming, Cellulite, Cleansing, Exfoliating, Healing, Insect Repellant, Itchy Skin, Lightening, Mature Skin, Moisturizing, Repairing, Scarring, Soothing

2 drops karanja oil or neem oil

3 drops lavender oil

3 drops tea tree oil or manuka oil

2 drops rosemary oil (optional)

2 Tablespoons milk

2 Tablespoons olive oil

Mix and soak infected area in this mixture with cotton pads. Wash off with warm water if you prefer. Great for tinea and ringworm

## ANTI-FUNGAL Yogurt, ROSEMARY, HONEY & LAVENDER REMEDY

Acne, Anti-aging Anti-fungal, Antiseptic, Antibacterial, Calming, Healing, Moisturizing, Soothing

5 drops lavender oil

½ cup Yogurt

1 Tablespoon honey

5 drops rosemary oil

Mix ingredients together and rub onto affected areas then rinse off after 10 minutes.

Acetylsalicylic acid (the chemical name for aspirin) is an anti-inflammatory. When applied to the skin, it will reduce inflammation and can also relieve pain. If you use powdered aspirin you'll also get the stimulating benefits of caffeine, which is great for skin.

½ Teaspoon aspirin powdered or tablets crushed

¼ Teaspoon of water

½ Teaspoon of oil (olive, almond, safflower of any other oil mentioned in this book will do)

½ Teaspoon of honey

Mix the ingredients together and apply to skin. Leave on for 10-20 minutes then rinse off with luke warm water.


## ANTI-INFLAMMATORY OIL BLEND

Anti-Septic, Anti-Bacterial, Anti-inflammatory, Moisturizer


10 drops rosehip oil

5 drops calophyllum oil

3 drops myrhh oil

10 drops almond oil

Blend oils together and rub in to affected areas as needed. Store in glass bottle.

## ANTI-INFLAMMATORY PEPPERMINT MUD MASK

Anti-aging, Anti-inflammatory, Discoloration, Insect Repellant

2 Tablespoons rubbing alcohol or vodka

1 Teaspoon peppermint extract

2 Teaspoon fuller's earth (clay)

Mix all ingredients together. Apply to face, avoiding eye area. Leave on for 10 minutes. Rinse off with warm water.

## ANTI-OXIDANT CALMING HOMEMADE FACIAL MASK WITH AUBERGINE

Anti-aging, Anti-inflammatory, Anti-oxidant, Balancing, Calming, Cleansing, Cooling, Exfoliating, Healing, Mature Skin, Moisturizing, Repairing, Repairing Acne, Scarring

2 oz aubergine (eggplant)

1 Teaspoon honey

2 Tablespoons St. John's Wort brew

1 Tablespoon aloe vera juice or gel

Wash and peel the eggplant then grate it into a blender. Blend or puree then add honey and other ingredients. Apply to skin and leave on for 10 minutes the wash off and repeat application, then rinsing off.

## ANTI-OXIDANT COFFEE COCONUT CHOCOLATE MASK

Anti-aging, Anti-bacterial, Anti-oxidant, Moisturizing

1 small chocolate bar

1 Teaspoon coconut oil

1 Tablespoon strong filtered coffee (espresso)

1 Teaspoon molasses if you want a glycolic peel effect with this mask

Instructions:

Melt these ingredients together and apply while warm to your skin. Leave on for ten minutes and wash off. This is rich in antioxidants and stimulates cell repair and regeneration.

## ANTI-OXIDANT EXFOLIATING APRICOT CREAM MASK

Acne, Anti-aging, Anti-fungal, Anti-inflammatory, Anti-oxidant, Brightening, Cleansing, Discoloration, Exfoliating, Insect Repellant, Lightening, Moisturizing, Soothing

1 cup dried apricots (soaked in water)

2 Tablespoons powdered milk

Soak Apricots in water until softened. Blend or puree apricots then add milk powder until combined into a smooth paste. Leave on for about 15 minutes then rinse off with warm water.

## ANTI-OXIDANT EXFOLIATING VITAMIN RICH FACIAL SCRUB

Age Spots, Anti-aging, Anti-oxidant, Exfoliating, Mature Skin, Moisturizing, Wrinkles

1 Teaspoon mint tea (steeped)

3 Tablespoons sunflower meal

1 fig

½ Tablespoon safflower oil

Cut a dry fig in half, dip one half in oil and mint tea mixture.

Rub it onto your clean washed face and gently massage to exfoliate. Rub in the leftover oil and leave to dry if you wish. Rinse off with the rest of the cold mint tea then pat dry with a cotton ball.

## ANTI-OXIDANT EXFOLIATOR ALMOND AND BERRY FACIAL MASK

Acne, Age Spots, Anti-aging, Anti-inflammatory, Anti-oxidant, Balancing, Brightening, Calming, Cleansing, Cooling, Dark Circles, Discoloration, Exfoliating, Healing, Lightening, Mature Skin, Moisturizing, Puffiness, Repairing, Scarring, Tightening

½ cucumber

1 Tablespoon yogurt

3 or 4 few berries

1 Teaspoon honey

In a food processor or blender, mix all ingredients together and apply to skin. Leave on for 10 minute and wash off with warm water.

## ANTI-OXIDANT RED WINE, CLAY AND POMEGRANATE MASK

Acne, Age Spots, Anti-aging, Anti-fungal, Anti-inflammatory, Anti-oxidant, Balancing, Brightening, Calming, Cleansing, Discoloration, Exfoliating, Healing, Lightening, Mature Skin, Moisturizing, Repairing, Scarring, Soothing

¼ pomegranate

1 Tablespoon red wine

3 Tablespoons rose clay (or plain clay with 3 drops or rose oil)

1 Tablespoon organic honey

½ Tablespoon coconut oil, coconut cream or finely ground coconut

Peel ¼ Pomegranate then cut and mash or puree it. Put the clay in a mixing bowl and slowly add the Pomegranate Coconut until it forms a paste.

Spread the paste gently and equally with your fingertips on your clean face and neck avoiding the eye area. Leave on for 15 minutes then wash off with warm water.

## ANTI-OXIDANT WATERMELON MASK

Cleansing, Anti-oxidant

2 slices of watermelon (remove the seeds) mashed

Mash water melon and squeeze juice out of the pulp using a strainer, coffee filter, muslin cloth, pantyhose or similar. Apply juice to face with cotton ball and rinse off after 10-15 minutes. You can add whipped cream or Yogurt for an extra moisturizing option.

## ANTI-OXIDANT YOGURT GREEN TEA & RED WINE TREATMENT

Anti-aging, Anti-inflammatory, Anti-oxidant, Calming, Cleansing, Exfoliating, Healing, Mature Skin, Moisturizing, Repairing, Scarring

1 Tablespoon green tea

1 Tablespoon red wine

1 Tablespoon plain Yogurt

2 Tablespoons organic honey

Make a cup of green tea and let it stand for a few minutes. Add the other ingredients and allow to cool until its cool enough to apply to your skin.

Apply and leave on for 15 minutes then wash off with warm water.

## ANTI-OXIDANT, AGE SPOTS, REJUVENATING PUMPKIN MASK

Acne, Age-spots, Anti-aging, Anti-fungal, Anti-inflammatory, Anti-oxidant, Brightening, Calming, Cleansing, Exfoliating, Healing, Lightening, Mature Skin, Moisturizing, Repairing, Scarring, Soothing, Tightening

½ cup fresh pumpkin pulp

2 eggs

2 Teaspoons almond milk (for dry or combo skin)

1 Teaspoon honey (for dry skin)

2 Teaspoons apple, cider vinegar or cranberry juice (if you have oily skin)

Purée the fresh Pumpkin pulp so it forms a thick paste. Add the egg as a binder. For dry skin add almond Milk and the Honey.  For oily complexions you can add apple, cranberry juice, lemon juice or apple cider vinegar. Blend well then apply to skin. Leave on for 15-20 minutes then rinse off with warm water.

## ANTIOXIDANT GRAPE TONIC FOR Sensitive Skin

Sensitive Skin, Anti-oxidant, Anti-inflammatory

Mash grapes and squeeze juice out of the pulp using a strainer, coffee filter, muslin cloth, pantyhose or similar. Apply juice to face with cotton ball and rinse off after 10-15 minutes. You can add whipped cream or Yogurt for an extra moisturizing option.

## ARROWROOT FACE MASK

Acne, Anti-aging, Anti-inflammatory, Anti-oxidant, Brightening, Calming, Cleansing, Exfoliating, Healing, Lightening, Mature Skin, Moisturizing, Repairing, Scarring, Soothing

1 oz fuller's earth

2 Teaspoons arrowroot

1 Teaspoon finely ground cornmeal

1 Teaspoon finely ground almond meal

Enough Honey, apple cider vinegar, or yogurt to form a soft paste.

Mix ingredients together, apply to skin and leave on for 10-15 minutes. Rinse with lukewarm water.

## BASIC CLAY MASK BASE (FOR ADDING OTHER "ACTIVE" INGREDIENTS & OILS TO)

Blackheads, Oily Skin, Moisturizing

2 oz green clay

3 Teaspoon cornflour

Mix ingredients together this base and store in a jar ready for adding oils and other ingredients to.  This is a good moisturizing clarifying base.

## BERGAMOT COLD CREAM

Acne, Anti-aging, Anti-fungal, Anti-inflammatory, Antibacterial, Antiseptic, Balancing, Calming, Cellulite, Cleansing, Discoloration, Insect Repellant, Mature Skin, Moisturizing, Soothing

½ Teaspoon borax powder

1 Tablespoon hot distilled water

½ cup almond oil

1 Tablespoon grated beeswax

1 Tablespoon rose flower water

2 drops bergamot oil

2 drops lavender oil

Mix borax powder and distilled water together for about half a minute. Add the Almond Oil and grated beeswax to a separate heatproof container and heat in a double boiler or microwave for two to three minutes on high so the beeswax is melted. Add rose flower water, Bergamot & lavender oils to the borax solution. Stir. Mix all of the ingredients together and blend for a couple of minutes until well combined and consistent in color.  Cool and store in glass of plastic containers.  Apply as needed.

## BODY SCRUBS

Mix one part of any oils listed in this book to one part sugar.  You can add other essential oils to scent the mix.  Mix well and apply to skin using hands or a loofah.  Rinse off with warm water.

## BODY & FACE HOME MADE BODY WAX

Exfoliating

3 Tablespoons sugar

3 Tablespoons lemon juice

1 Tablespoon water

Cook over low heat until the sugar caramelizes into a gooey mixture. After cooling it should form a sticky taffy-like wax.  Apply with a plastic knife or wooden stick in the direction hair grows. Take a piece of cloth, press down firmly and then pull off in the opposite direction of hair growth.

## BRIGHTENING BANANA CHICKPEA MASK

Cleansing, Exfoliating, Tightening, Stimulating

1 ripe banana peeled and mashed

4 Tablespoons chickpea flour (or cooked mashed chickpeas)

1 egg beaten

Mix the ingredients together and apply to skin.  Leave on for 10-20 minutes then rinse off with luke warm water.

## BRIGHTENING MASK FOR ASHY SKIN

Cleansing, Exfoliating, Moisturizing

2 Tablespoons sugar

3 Tablespoons warm water

Mix the ingredients together and rub gently onto skin avoiding the delicate eye areas. Rinse off with luke warm water.

## BRIGHTENING AND MOISTURIZING ALOE VERA MASK

Balancing, Brightening, Moisturizing, Soothing

½ cup aloe vera juice

Pinch salt

Mix ingredients together and apply to skin with cotton pad for tightening and balancing skin.

## BRIGHTENING STIMULATING COCOA AND COFFEE MASK

Acne, Anti-aging, Anti-fungal, Anti-inflammatory, Anti-oxidant, Balancing, Brightening, Calming, Cellulite, Cleansing, Discoloration, Exfoliating, Healing, Insect Repellant, Lightening, Mature Skin, Moisturizing, Repairing, Scarring, Soothing

4 Tablespoons finely ground espresso or coffee beans

4 Tablespoons unsweetened cocoa powder

8 Tablespoons dairy product (milk, plain yogurt, almond milk or coconut milk).

If you like a thicker paste you can use an egg instead of dairy, or substitute oils, such as Olive Oil, extra virgin Coconut if you have dehydrated skin. If using oils, you will need to halve the amount or it will be too runny.

2 Tablespoons Honey (for dry skin) or lemon juice (for oily skin)

Mix coffee and cocoa powder in a bowl. Add other ingredients then apply to skin.

Let the mask dry before washing off. Store any leftover paste in the refrigerator for up to 6 days.


## BRIGHTENING VITAMIN C SERUM FOR EVEN SKIN TONE AND SCAR REDUCTION

Balancing, Brightening, Discoloration, Moisturizing, Scarring, Soothing


5 tablespoons Rose hip oil

1 teaspoon Avocado oil

4 drops of Carrot seed oil

Blend these oils together and store out of direct sunlight in a coolish place. Store in a glass bottle preferably or used cleanser bottle.

Apply once or twice daily for a very rich rejuvenating anti aging skin serum.


## CALMING ACNE APPLE FACE MASK

Acne, Anti-aging, Anti-oxidant, Brightening, Calming, Cleansing, Exfoliating, Healing, Itchy Skin, Lightening, Moisturizing, Scarring, Soothing, Tightening


2 apples, peeled and mashed

1 Teaspoon of Jojoba Oil

1 Tablespoon Chamomile tea

Mix the ingredients together.  Apply to the face and leave on for 10 minutes. Rinse off with warm water.

## CARROT FACIAL MASK

Anti-aging, Anti-inflammatory, Anti-oxidant, Calming, Cleansing, Exfoliating, Healing, Mature Skin, Moisturizing, Repairing, Scarring

2-3 large cooked mashed carrots

4 ½ Tablespoons honey

Mix the ingredients together and apply to skin.  Leave on for 10-20 minutes then rinse off with luke warm water.

## CELLULITE SMOOTHER

Anti-aging, Anto-oxidant, Cellulite, Exfoliating, Repairing, Mature Skin, Moisturizing

½ cup hazelnut, apricot, coconut or almond oil

4 drops lavender oil

6 drops grapefruit oil

5 drops rosemary oil

5 drops geranium oil

½ Teaspoon orange, lemon or lime juice

5 drops frankincense oil

4 drops ginger oil or 10 drops ginger (squeezed) juice

4 drops juniper oil (optional)

Alternative oils for cellulite are listed under the cellulite category and the oils above can be substituted with those.

Blend together and apply to affected areas. This is a great cellulite blend that can be made into a cream with the addition of 2 Tablespoon beeswax melted with base oil before adding essential oils to the mix.

## CLEANSING ACNE MASK

Anti-aging, Anti-inflammatory, Anti-oxidant, Balancing, Calming, Cleansing, Discoloration, Exfoliating, Healing, Insect Repellant, Mature Skin, Moisturizing, Repairing, Scarring

1 Teaspoon green clay

1 Teaspoon liquid honey

1 Teaspoon yogurt or sour cream

1 drop geranium oil

Mix ingredients together all the ingredients together and apply to skin. Leave on for 10-15 minutes then rinse off with warm water.

## CLEANSING APRICOT BUTTER CREAM

Acne, Anti-aging, Anti-inflammatory, Balancing, Cleansing, Discoloration, Healing, Insect Repellant, Itchy Skin, Mature Skin, Moisturizing, Scarring, Wrinkles

10 oz apricot kernel oil

2 oz cocoa butter

2 oz beeswax

Melt all ingredients together using a double boiler until wax and butter are soft enough to combine. Beat until smooth and cooled. Pour into glass of plastic containers and use as needed.

## CLEANSING MOISTURIZING BASE CREAM

Anti-aging, Cleansing, Dry Skin, Mature Skin, Moisturizing

½ oz beeswax

1 oz lanolin (hydrous)

1 oz grapeseed oil

2 oz almond oil

1 oz avocado oil

3 oz distilled water,

2 drops clary sage oil

2 drops lemon oil

2 drops lavender oil

Melt oil, lanolin and beeswax together in a double boiler, cool a little then add essential oils of your choice.  Next slowly whisk in water until mixture has cooled.  Store in glass of plastic jars out of direct sunlight. This is a very nourishing moisturizing cream that you can add other essential oils to that suit your specific skin type and condition.

* To make this an exfoliating cleanser, add ground almonds, ground oatmeal, ground sunflower seeds or brown sugar to this mix just before applying to your skin.

## COOLING MELON COOLER SALT SCRUB

Acne, Anti-oxidant, Balancing, Calming, Cooling, Exfoliating, Moisturizing, Repairing

½ cup fine sea salt

1 oz aloe vera oil

½ oz watermelon seed oil or watermelon flesh

1 Tablespoon Carrot Root Powder or 3 drops carrot seed oil

1 Teaspoon menthol crystals (crushed) or almond meal or sunflower meal

2 Tablespoons cantaloupe

Mix all ingredients together and massage gently onto skin in a circular motion. Rinse off with warm water.

## COOLING REFRESHING FACIAL BUTTER RECIPE

Anti-aging, Balancing, Cleansing, Mature Skin, Moisturizing,

½ cup olive, coconut or almond oil

½ cup beeswax

1 ¼ cups of water

Emulsifying wax

Alpha lipoic acid powder

Combine wax and oil into a bowl sitting in a double boiler or saucepan filled with water. Heat the beeswax and oil until melted then stir together.  Fill a 2 cup measuring cup halfway with boiling water. Pour the combined melted wax and oil into the hot water, and gently whisk until it reaches the consistency of Milk and of consistent color. Stir in 2

Teaspoons of the alpha lipoic acid mixing well. While hot and runny pour into containers. You an add 4 to 8 drops of your favorite essential oils like lemon, neroli, tangerine or Lavender to the moisturizer mixture before the final cooling and mixing stage if you wish. Store in a cool place out of direct sunlight. Apply as needed.

## DARK CIRCLES BALM

Acne, Age Spots, Anti-oxidant, Balancing, Brightening, Calming, Cooling, Dark Circles, Discoloration, Healing, Itchy Skin, Lightening, Puffiness, Scarring, Soothing, Tightening

1 Tablespoon cucumber

Pinch gelatin (½ Teaspoon)

Chamomile tea (teabag infused in half a cup of water)

Mix ingredients together while tea infusion is still warm, allow to cool, then apply twice a day gently by patting around eye area with fingertips or cotton pad. Don't drag skin. This recipe is a great circle remover You can also use Cucumber directly as a skin treatment.

## DRY SKIN AVOCADO TREATMENT

Anti-aging, Anti-inflammatory, Anti-oxidant, Antibacterial, Antiseptic, Calming, Cleansing, Exfoliating, Healing, Mature Skin, Moisturizing, Repairing, Scarring, Wrinkles

½ an avocado

½ cup honey

Mash the avocado then Mix the ingredients together and apply to skin. Leave on for 10-20 minutes then rinse off with luke warm water.

## DRY SKIN BASIC MASK

Dry Skin, Blackheads, Moisturizing

2 oz green clay

3 Teaspoons cornflour

1 egg yolk

1 Teaspoon almond, wheatgerm or evening primrose oil

2 drops carrot oil

2 Teaspoons water or honey

1 drop rose oil

Combine all together and apply to skin. Leave on for 10 minutes then rinse off with warm water.

## DRY SKIN STRAWBERRY FACE MASK

Anti-aging, Anti-inflammatory, Discoloration

3 or 4 strawberries (mashed)

1 Teaspoon of butter or whipped cream

Mix the ingredients together. Apply to the face and leave on for 10 minutes. Rinse off with warm water.

## ECZEMA EGG WHITE AND POTATO MASK

Irritated Skin, Wrinkles, Lightening, Oily Skin, Tightening

1 small potato

1 egg white

2-3 drops carrot seed oil essential oil

Peel and grate the potato then mix with one egg white and the drops of carrot seed oil.

Smooth onto the skin and allow to dry. Rinse with warm water.


## EDIBLE SOOTHING CHOCOLATE MASK

Anti-aging, Anti-inflammatory, Anti-oxidant, Balancing, Calming, Cleansing, Discoloration, Exfoliating, Healing, Insect Repellant, Itchy Skin, Mature Skin, Moisturizing, Repairing, Scarring, Soothing


3 or 4 Tablespoons raw dark cacao powder

3 Tablespoons organic honey or manuka honey

4 Tablespoons organic yogurt or heavy cream

3 Tablespoons powdered oatmeal

Mix all ingredients together to form a thick paste and apply to face leaving on for 10 minutes before rinsing off with warm water.


## EXFOLIATING ANTI-OXIDANT PINEAPPLE FACE MASK

Anti-aging, Cleansing, Exfoliating, Healing, Mature Skin, Moisturizing, Repairing, Scarring


2 Teaspoons of chopped pineapple fresh (or tinned no added sugar variety)

3 Teaspoons of extra virgin olive oil

Blend all ingredients together forming a soft puree, apply to skin and leave on for no longer then 10 minutes. Wash off with warm water.

## EXFOLIATING CITRUS MASK

Acne, Anti-aging, Anti-oxidant, Blackheads, Cleansing, Discoloration, Exfoliating, Healing, Mature Skin, Moisturizing, Oily Skin, Repairing, Scarring, Tightening

1 Tablespoon gotu kola

2 Tablespoons green tea or loose leaf tea (brewed or steeped)

1 Tablespoon plain yogurt

1 Tablespoon grapeseed or olive oil

1-5 drops sweet orange oil

Mix the Gotu Kola and 1-5 drops of the essential oil to the Grapeseed or Olive Oil.

Massage into your face. Allow to sit o your skin for as long as you like then rinse off with warm water.

## EXFOLIATING COFFEE AND PLUM PASTE

Anti-inflammatory, Anti-oxidant, Calming, Cleansing, Exfoliating, Healing, Mature Skin, Moisturizing, Repairing, Scarring, Stimulating

2 Tablespoons ground coffee

3 plums crushed (or enough to mix with coffee to a paste)

Mix the ingredients together and apply to skin. Leave on for 10 minutes then rinse off with luke warm water.

## EXFOLIATOR ALPHA HYDROXY SKIN PEEL RECIPE

Anti-aging, Anti-inflammatory, Anti-oxidant, Calming, Cleansing, Exfoliating, Healing, Mature Skin, Moisturizing, Repairing, Scarring

1 cup fresh pineapple

½ cup fresh papaya

2 Tablespoons honey

Puree pineapple and papaya in a blender or similar. Add Honey and mix thoroughly.

Apply the mixture to your skin, avoiding the eye area. Leave on for no more than 5 minutes (less if you have Sensitive Skin), then rinse off with warm water.

## EXFOLIATOR BASIC SCRUB RECIPE FOR FACIAL EXFOLIATING

Dry Skin, Exfoliator, Mature Skin, Moisturizing, Soothing

1 Tablespoon ground almonds

1 Teaspoon ground oatmeal

½ Teaspoon cider vinegar or water and fruit juice mixed together ½ and ½

Enough oil (olive, almond, wheatgerm, coconut, apricot etc) to make a paste.

Apply to skin in a gentle circular motion then rinse off with warm water.

## EXFOLIATOR BROWN SUGAR MOISTURIZING HAND SCRUB

Acne, Anti-aging, Anti-fungal, Anti-inflammatory, Balancing, Brightening, Cellulite, Cleansing, Exfoliating, Lightening, Mature Skin, Moisturizing, Soothing

¼ cup brown sugar

3 Tablespoons milk

1 drop almond oil

Heat over low heat until a paste forms. Add Almond Oil, stirring in and allow to cool. Spread on hands, leave on for about 10 minutes, then gently scrub. Rinse off with warm water.

## EXFOLIATOR EDIBLE ALMOND MEAL SCRUB

Acne, Anti-aging, Anti-fungal, Anti-inflammatory, Anti-oxidant, Brightening, Calming, Cleansing, Exfoliating, Healing, Lightening, Mature Skin, Moisturizing, Repairing, Scarring, Soothing

2 Teaspoons milk (powdered or fresh)

½ Tablespoon honey

2 Tablespoons finely ground almonds

½ Teaspoon chickpea flour (besan)

Mix ingredients together well and apply to face rubbing in a gentle circular motion. Wait for 10-15 minutes and rinse off with warm water.

## EYE SERUM 20'S & 30'S

2 Teaspoons hazelnut or almond oil

2 drops borage oil

1 vitamin E capsule

4 drops evening primrose oil

2 drops lavender oil

3 drops carrot seed oil

1 drop lemon or orange oil

Add 3 drops fennel if you have dark circles under your eyes

Blend and store out of direct sunlight in a glass eye dropper bottle preferably. Apply gently by dabbing around the eye area. Do not rub or pull the skin around your eyes.


## EYE SERUM 40'S AND 50'S

2 Teaspoons hazelnut or almond oil

2 drops borage oil

5 drops jojoba oil

4 drops rosehip oil

1 vitamin E capsule

4 drops evening primrose oil

2 drops lavender oil

3 drops carrot seed oil

1 drop lemon or orange oil

Add 3 drops fennel if you have dark circles under your eyes

Blend and store out of direct sunlight in a glass eye dropper bottle preferably. Apply gently by dabbing around the eye area. Do not rub or pull the skin around your eyes.

## FOOT SOAK BLEND

2 Tablespoons almond oil

4 drops peppermint oil

4 drops tea tree oil

2 drops lavender and/or rosemary oil

Add these ingredients to a foot soak for a relaxing refreshing and deodorizing treat.

## HEALING CALENDULA OINTMENT

Acne, Anti-aging, Anti-inflammatory, Balancing, Calming, Cleansing, Healing, Mature Skin, Moisturizing, Repairing, Scarring, Soothing

2 cups of dried calendula flowers or 10 drops calendula oil

3 cups of coconut oil

2 ½ cups beeswax

10 drops of essential oil for scenting your ointment

Heat Calendula with the Coconut and beeswax for 90 minutes in a double boiler if using calendula flowers or 20 minutes if using calendula oil. Blend in essential oil and sieve through muslin cloth, a coffee filter or tea towel set in a wire mesh strainer.

Apply to wounds as a preventative for scarring or to existing scars to reduce scar tissue.

## HEALING CALENDULA SERUM

Acne, Anti-aging, Anti-inflammatory, Balancing, Calming, Cleansing, Healing, Mature Skin, Moisturizing, Repairing, Scarring, Soothing

2 tablespoons Almond oil (can also make a mix of Argan, Almond and/or Wheatgerm oils for a richer blend but I have said Almond oil here as it's the easiest to find)

1 teaspoon Rosehip oil (optional but this oil is excellent for scars and stretch marks)

4 drops Calendula oil

4 drops Carrot seed oil

3 drops Borage oil (optional but makes it more potent for better results)

Blend together well by shaking in a glass bottle. Store in a cool place out of direct sunlight. Apply a few drops daily (or twice daily if you wish) to a clean face under moisturizer. It is also nice applied to the décolletage – an area many people forget to look after.

This is a beautifully light blend but delivers lots of benefits deep into your skin's layers.

## ITCHY SKIN MOISTURIZING ANTI-AGING OIL BLEND

Acne, Anti-aging, Anti-fungal, Anti-inflammatory, Anti-oxidant, Antibacterial, Antiseptic, Balancing, Brightening, Calming, Cleansing, Healing, Insect Repellant, Itchy Skin, Lightening, Moisturizing, Repairing, Scarring, Soothing, SPF Protection, Wrinkles

24 drops apricot kernel oil

7 drops chamomile oil

4 drops karanja oil

4 drops manuka oil

5 drops neem oil

10 drops wheat germ oil

Mix these oils together and massage into skin. Allow to absorb into your skin for a few minutes, then apply your favorite moisturizer or foundation.

## LIGHTENING/BRIGHTENING OIL BLEND

Acne, Age Spots, Anti-aging, Anti-inflammatory, Anti-oxidant, Balancing, Brightening, Calming, Cellulite, Cleansing, Discoloration, Healing, Itchy Skin, Lightening, Mature Skin, Moisturizing, Repairing, Scarring, Soothing

7 drops chamomile oil

10 drops rosehip oil

Mix these oils together and massage into skin.

## LIP GLOSS

1 oz beeswax

2 Tablespoons sweet almond oil, safflower or light olive oil

10 drops jojoba oil

3 drops olive oil (optional)

5 drops carrot seed oil

Heat beeswax and almond oil in a double boiler until melted. Add other oils and blend until smooth. Store in lip gloss sized containers.

## MACADAMIA NIGHTLY FACIAL FOR DRY SKIN

Anti-aging, Mature Skin, Moisturizing, Wrinkles

6 Teaspoons macadamia nut oil

2 Teaspoons hydrous Lanolin

2 Teaspoons beeswax

4 Teaspoons rose hydrosol or 3 drops rose oil

4 Teaspoons aloe vera gel or juice (optional)

⅛ Teaspoon borax powder

8 drops rose essential oil

1 drop benzoin essential oil

Put the oil, Lanolin and beeswax in a double boiler heating until the wax melts. Heat the hydrosol and aloe in a separate pan. Next add the borax powder and stir until dissolved. Slowly add the hydrosol mixing as you go until the mixture forms into a cream. Allow to cool slightly then add essential oil. Once cools fill clean plastic or glass jars with mixture and store inn a cool dark place.

## MAKEUP REMOVER CASTOR OIL BLEND

Anti-aging, Cleansing, Healing, Mature Skin, Moisturizing, Repairing, Scarring

1 Tablespoon castor oil

1 Tablespoon olive oil

Blend oils together. Apply oil to a cotton ball or q-tip and swipe off the make-up.

## MATURE SKIN OIL BLEND

Acne, Age Spots, Anti-aging, Anti-fungal, Anti-inflammatory, Anti-oxidant, Antibacterial, Antiseptic, Balancing, Brightening, Cellulite, Cleansing, Discoloration, Exfoliating, Healing, Lightening, Mature Skin, Moisturizing, Repairing, Scarring, Soothing, Tightening, Wrinkles

24 drops almond oil

5 drops argan oil

10 drops avocado oil

6 drops carrot seed oil

5 drops clary sage oil

24 drops coconut oil

10 drops evening primrose oil

3 drops frankincense oil

10 drops macadamia oil (optional)

10 drops olive oil

10 drops rosehip oil

15 drops safflower oil

8 drops borage oil

Mix these oils together and massage into skin.

## MOISTURIZING ACNE SUNFLOWER ARTICHOKE FACIAL

Acne, Age Spots, Anti-aging, Anti-oxidant, Moisturizing

1 fresh artichoke heart well cooked or canned hearts in water (not oil)

2 Teaspoons light sunflower oil

1 Teaspoon vinegar or fresh lemon juice

Mash, blend or puree artichoke. Mix in all the ingredients together and apply to skin. Leave on for 10-15 minutes then rinse off with warm water.

## MOISTURIZING BANANA CREAM TREATMENT

Acne, Anti-aging, Anti-fungal, Anti-inflammatory, Anti-oxidant, Brightening, Cleansing, Discoloration, Exfoliating, Insect Repellant, Lightening, Moisturizing, Soothing, Tightening

1 capsule of Vitamin E

1 ripe banana peeled and mashed

¼ cup of heavy whipping cream

Mix the ingredients together and apply to skin. Leave on for 10-20 minutes then rinse off with luke warm water.

## MOISTURIZING BANANA FACIAL MASK

Anti-aging, Anti-inflammatory, Anti-oxidant, Calming, Cleansing, Discoloration and Honey, Discoloration Anti-aging, Exfoliating, Healing, Insect Repellant, Mature Skin, Moisturizing, Repairing, Repairing, Scarring, Tightening

½ banana mashed

1 Tablespoon honey

2 Tablespoons sour cream

Mix ingredients together, apply to skin and leave on for about 10 minutes. Rinse off with warm water.

## MOISTURIZING COCONUT CREAM AVOCADO MASK

Acne, Anti-aging, Anti-fungal, Anti-inflammatory, Anti-oxidant, Cleansing, Moisturizing

1 Tablespoon coconut cream or oil

1/2 a mashed avocado

Mix well and apply to skin then wash off after ten to 15 minutes. Add essential oils if you wish for anti aging or to reduce lines and wrinkles or even red veins. If you have scars add some rose hip and carrot seed oil.

## MOISTURIZING PROTECTIVE COCONUT OIL FACE MASK

Anti-aging, Anti-inflammatory, Anti-oxidant, Balancing, Calming, Cleansing, Exfoliating, Healing, Mature Skin, Moisturizing, Repairing, Scarring

½ cup coconut oil

1 Teaspoon honey

Blend ingredients together and apply to skin. Leave the mask on for 10 minutes, then rinse off with warm water.

## MOISTURIZING EXFOLIATING MASK

Anti-aging, Balancing, Cleansing, Exfoliating, Healing, Mature Skin, Moisturizing, Moisturizing oil, Repairing, Scarring

1 Tablespoon brown sugar

1 Teaspoon (more or less, add drops if you need them) of Olive Oil or extra virgin Coconut oil

Mix into a paste then massage into skin in a circular motion.  Rinse off with warm water.

## MOISTURIZING FACIAL TREATMENT OIL

Acne, Anti-aging, Anti-inflammatory, Antibacterial, Antiseptic, Balancing, Brightening, Cellulite, Cleansing, Lightening, Mature Skin, Moisturizing, Soothing

1 oz coconut oil

1 oz sweet almond oil

10 drops juniper oil

7 drops vanilla essential oil (can use neroil, bergamot or rose oils)

Put the bottle in a cool, dark place, and let the mixture infuse for 72 hours before the first use.

Blend ingredients in a glass bottle shaking well.  Massage into skin before applying make-up in the mornings or after a facial treatment.

## MOISTURIZING GHASSOUL CLAY & ARGAN OIL FACIAL MASK

Anti-oxidant, Mature Skin, Moisturizing

½ Tablespoon moroccan ghassoul powder

½ Teaspoon argan oil

½ Teaspoon almond oil

Combine mixture together and apple to skin. Apply and leave on for a maximum of 5 minutes. Rinse off with warm water.

## MOISTURIZING LANOLIN FACIAL NIGHT CREAM GEL

Acne, Anti-aging, Anti-inflammatory, Balancing, Calming, Cleansing, Cooling, Discoloration, Healing, Insect Repellant, Itchy Skin, Mature Skin, Moisturizing, Repairing, Scarring, Tightening, Wrinkles

1 Tablespoon aloe vera

⅛ cup distilled water

1 Tablespoon beeswax (white)

⅛ cup lanolin (anhydrous)

3 drops frankincense oil

1 drops lemon essential oil

⅛ cup 2 Teaspoons jojoba oil (cold pressed)

⅛ cup 2 Teaspoons apricot kernel oil

Add the aloe gel to the oil and whisk to mix thoroughly. Set aside. In a double boiler, heat beeswax and Lanolin until just melted. Stir in aloe oil and distilled water and keep stirring until mixture thickens. Add mixture to jars and lightly cap until mixture completely cools then tighten caps. Apply to face every evening.

## MOISTURIZING NEROLI AND LICORICE FACIAL SCRUB

Acne, Anti-aging, Anti-fungal, Anti-inflammatory, Balancing, Brightening, Cellulite, Cleansing, Discoloration, Exfoliating, Healing, Insect Repellant, Itchy Skin, Lightening, Mature Skin, Moisturizing, Scarring, Soothing

½ cup finely ground almonds

1 Tablespoon ground oatmeal (can grind or blend oatmeal or almonds together)

2 Tablespoon soured milk, sour cream or Yogurt

2 drops of neroli

1 drop of licorice root extract

1 Tablespoon almond oil

Grind almonds and Oatmeal in a blender to a fine pulp or powder. Add soured Milk to bond the mixture. Add licorice root extract, Neroli and Almond Oils. Apply to face in a gentle rubbing motion avoiding the eye area. Leave on for 10 minutes then rinse off with warm water.

## MOISTURIZING OATMEAL, BALANCING, ITCHY SKIN, SOOTHING FACE MASK

Acne, Anti-fungal, Balancing, Brightening, Cleansing, Exfoliating, Itchy Skin, Lightening, Moisturizing, Soothing, Tightening

1 ripe mashed banana

1 cup of ground oatmeal

Mix the ingredients together and apply to skin then rub to exfoliate skin. Leave on for 10-20 minutes then rinse off with luke warm water.

## MOISTURIZING OIL BLEND

Acne, Age Spots, Anti-aging, Anti-fungal, Anti-inflammatory, Anti-oxidant, Antibacterial, Antifungal, Antiseptic, Balancing, Brightening, Cellulite, Cleansing, Discoloration, Exfoliating, Healing, Itchy Skin, Lightening, Mature Skin, Moisturizing, Moisturizing, Repairing, Scarring, Soothing, Tightening, Wrinkles

6 drops carrot seed oil

10 drops olive oil

4 drops clary sage oil

24 drops coconut oil

10 drops evening primrose oil

3 drops frankincense oil

24 drops grape seed oil

4 drops hazelnuts oil

24 drops jojoba oil

3 drops juniper oil

10 drops macadamia oil

24 drops almond oil

24 drops apricot kernel oil

5 drops argan oil

10 drops avocado oil

5 drops flax seed oil

## MOISTURIZING ROSE HIP FACE MASK

Anti-aging, Anti-inflammatory, Anti-oxidant, Balancing, Calming, Cleansing, Exfoliating, Healing, Mature Skin, Moisturizing, Repairing, Scarring

1 Tablespoon white clay

3 drops of rose hip oil

½ Teaspoon honey

4 drops rose geranium

Mix ingredients together all the ingredients together and apply to skin. Leave on for 10-15 minutes then rinse off with warm water.

## MOISTURIZING SOOTHING FACE MASK

Acne, Anti-fungal, Brightening, Exfoliating, Lightening, Moisturizing, Soothing

1 bar dark chocolate

3 Tablespoon salt

1 cup milk

Melt the chocolate (preferably in a double boiler) then add other. Apply to face and leave on for 15 minutes then rinse off with warm water.

## MOISTURIZING, ANTI-OXIDANT CUCUMBER KIWI MASK

Acne, Age Spots, Anti-aging, Anti-fungal, Anti-inflammatory, Anti-oxidant, Antibacterial, Antiseptic, Balancing, Brightening, Calming, Cellulite, Cleansing, Cooling, Dark Circles, Discoloration, Exfoliating, Insect Repellant, Lightening, Puffiness, Soothing, Tightening

2 oz fresh cucumber

½ kiwi fruit peeled

1 Teaspoon fresh whipping cream

1 Tablespoon finely powdered oats

1 Tablespoon kaolin clay

4 drops lavender oil

Mix or blend all ingredients together Store unused portion in the fridge for a few days

## NATURAL INSECT REPELLING SPF FACIAL & BODY OIL

Anti-aging, Anti-fungal, Anti-inflammatory, Antibacterial, Antiseptic, Balancing, Calming, Cellulite, Cleansing, Mature Skin, Moisturizing, Soothing

5 drops neem oil

5 drops karanja oil

5 drops sesame oil

3 drops sandalwood oil

4 drops lavender oil or sandalwood, neroli, ylang ylang or rose oils

2 Tablespoons sweet almond oil

2 Tablespoons coconut oil

Combine no more then 2-10% neem and Karanja Oil with sesame oil, sweet Almond Oil, & coconut oil. Add any essential oils like Lavender or sandalwood oils.

Apply to face, neck and other exposed areas before going outside in the elements.

## NORMAL SKIN BASIC MASK

Balancing, Moisturizing, Repairing

2 oz green clay

3 Teaspoons cornflour

1 egg yolk

1 Teaspoon water

1 drop geranium oil

1 drop bergamot oil

Combine all together and apply to skin. Leave on for 10 minutes then rinse off with warm water.

## NORMAL SKIN CLEANSING CLAY MASK

Acne, Balancing, Cooling, Calming, Moisturizing, Repairing

1½ Teaspoon green clay

½ Teaspoon kaolin clay

1½ Tablespoon aloe vera gel

1 Tablespoon rosewater

2 drops rose essential oil

Mix the ingredients together and apply to skin. Leave on for 10-20 minutes then rinse off with luke warm water.

Refrigerate mixture for up to one month.

## NORMAL SKIN EGG WHITE YOGURT MASK

Anti-aging, Blackheads, Brightening, Cleansing, Lightening, Oily Skin, Tightening, Wrinkles

2 egg whites

2 Tablespoons plain yogurt

Mix the ingredients together and apply to skin. Leave on for 10-20 minutes then rinse off with luke warm water.

## NORMAL SKIN PUMPKIN FACIAL FOR ANY SKIN TYPE

Acne, Age-spots, Anti-aging, Anti-inflammatory, Anti-oxidant, Calming, Cleansing, Discoloration, Exfoliating, Healing, Insect Repellant, Mature Skin, Moisturizing, Repairing, Scarring, Tightening

Tablespoon cooked pumpkin mashed

1 Tablespoon honey

**For Dry Skin**

¼ Teaspoon heavy whipping cream

½ Teaspoon brown sugar

**For Oily Skin**

¼ Teaspoon Apple cider or apple cider vinegar

¼ Teaspoon cranberry juice

Mix well and apply all over your face. Leave for about 10-15 minutes then rinse off with warm water.

## NORMAL SKIN STIMULATING MOISTURIZING MASK

Anti-aging, Lightening, Moisturizing, Wrinkles

1 Tablespoon turmeric powder

1 cup of plain yogurt

Mix the ingredients together and apply to skin. Leave on for 10-20 minutes then rinse off with luke warm water.

## NOURISHING MASK FOR COMBINATION SKIN

Acne, Anti-fungal, Anti-oxidant, Antibacterial, Antiseptic, Balancing, Calming, Cellulite, Cleansing, Exfoliating, Itchy Skin, Mature Skin, Moisturizing, Rejuvenating, Renewing, Repairing, Soothing, Tightening, Wrinkles

½ cup oatmeal

½ an avocado

1 inch chunk of papaya (you can substitute papaya for strawberries or blueberries)

1 inch strip of aloe vera gel or juice

2 drops of eucalyptus oil

2 drops of lavender oil

Blend the Oatmeal to a fine pulp and then add papaya (or berries) and aloe. Add a touch of filtered water if the mixture is too dry. Next add essential oils. Leave on the face for about 15 minutes then rinse off with warm water.

## OILY SKIN & ALOE JUICE

Apply aloe juice with cotton pad daily. For oily or combination skin add a few drops of lemon juice to the mix. Allow to dry then rinse with water. This mask is also very effective for overall skin improvement, brightening and moisturizing.

Tip: To reduce oil production you can simply apply freshly squeezed aloe juice to your face twice a day (morning and evening). Store aloe in the fridge for around 2 weeks before use to intensify concentration of biologically active and make the juice extraction process easier.

## OILY SKIN APPLE MASK

Acne, Anti-oxidant, Cleansing, Exfoliating, Moisturizing, Tightening

1 apple peeled and mashed or pureed

1 egg yolk

Mix well, apply to the skin, leave on for 10 minutes then rinse off with warm water.

## OILY SKIN AVOCADO MASK

Anti-oxidant, Antibacterial, Antiseptic, Mature Skin, Moisturizing, Repairing, Wrinkles

1 egg white

1 Teaspoon lemon juice

½ an avocado

Mix the ingredients together in a blender and apply to skin. Leave on for 10-20 minutes then rinse off with luke warm water.

## OILY SKIN BALANCING COMBINATION SKIN MASK

Anti-aging, Anti-inflammatory, Anti-oxidant, Calming, Cleansing, Exfoliating, Healing, Mature Skin, Moisturizing, Repairing, Scarring


Optional: 6 fresh rose petals

2 Tablespoons rosewater

1 Tablespoon natural yogurt, room temperature (not low fat or non-fat)

1 Tablespoon runny (warmed) Honey

Soak rose petals, then crush them in a bowl or mortar & pestle.  Mix the ingredients together and apply to skin.  Leave on for 15 minutes then rinse off with luke warm water.


## OILY SKIN BANANA EGG WHITE MASK

Anti-aging, Age Spots, Cleansing, Discoloration, Exfoliating, Lightening, Tightening


1 mashed banana

1 Teaspoon of lemon juice

1 egg yolk

Mix the ingredients together and apply to skin.  Leave on for 10-20 minutes then rinse off with luke warm water.

## OILY SKIN BANANA MASK

Cleansing, Exfoliating, Anti-oxidant, Lightening, Tightening


1 banana mashed

1 Teaspoon of lemon juice

1 egg yolk

Mix ingredients together and apply to skin.  Leave on for 10 minutes then rinse off with warm water.


## OILY SKIN BASIC MASK

2 oz green clay or white clay

3 Teaspoon cornflour

1 Tablespoon brewers yeast or almond meal

1 Tablespoon water

1 drop rosemary oil

1 drop lavender oil

1 drop tea tree oil if you have problem acneic skin

Combine all together and apply to skin.  Leave on for 10 minutes then rinse off with warm water.


## OILY SKIN CAT LITTER MASK

Acne, Blackheads, Oily Skin

Bentonite clay is one of the natural clays found in expensive spa facials. Many cat/kitty litters are made of the same clay dried.  You can use cat litter & check the  for "sodium bentonite clay" or "100 percent natural

clay."

1 bag cat litter (must be marked as above)

A little water, enough to form a smooth paste

A few drops of your favorite essential oil

Mix in a couple Tablespoon the cat litter with water and drops of oil to smooth out the mixture and make it less coarse. Apply mask to face then wash off after 15 minutes with warm water.


## OILY SKIN COTTAGE CHEESE MASK

Acne, Anti-fungal, Brightening, Exfoliating, Lightening, Moisturizing, Soothing


2 Teaspoons low fat cottage cheese

2 Teaspoons tomato crushed, or carrot juice or strawberries crushed

Pinch of sea salt

Mix the ingredients together and apply to skin. Leave on for 10-20 minutes then rinse off with luke warm water. Repeat a second time for best results.


## OILY SKIN EXFOLIATOR JUICE

Anti-aging, Anti-oxidant, Cleansing, Exfoliator, Tightening, Wrinkles


⅓ cup papaya juice or combination of papaya and pineapple juices

Apply to the face, neck or hands with a cloth or cotton ball. Remove after a maximum of 10 minutes no longer as this is a powerful exfoliator.

## OILY SKIN FENNEL STEAM FACIAL

Acne, Anti-oxidant, Antibacterial, Antiseptic, Cleansing, Exfoliating, Moisturizing, Red Veins, Tightening

2 Teaspoons fennel seeds or 3 drops fennel oil

1 Teaspoon dried parsley

2 cup distilled water

2 Tablespoons witch hazel or apple coder vinegar

Towel

Small container with a lid

Add the Fennel and Parsley to the water in a wide-mouthed pot. Bring to a boil. Remove the pot from the heat. Immediately drape your head with the towel and lean over the steam – keeping yourself far away enough that you don't burn your skin. Allow the steam to mist your face for at least five minutes. Dry with a soft cloth.

## OILY SKIN HONEY AND PAPAYA MASK

Anti-aging, Anti-inflammatory, Anti-oxidant, Balancing, Calming, Cleansing, Discoloration, Exfoliating, Healing, Itchy Skin, Mature Skin, Moisturizing, Repairing, Scarring, Soothing

2 Tablespoons cocoa

3 Teaspoons of heavy cream

2 Tablespoons ripe papaya pulp

2 Teaspoons of honey

3 Teaspoons of oatmeal powder (ground oatmeal).

Mix ingredients together carefully and apply to the face to 10-15 minutes after which wash off with warm water. This anti aging mask is good for blemishes, greasy and acne-prone skin

## OILY SKIN MILK OATMEAL MASK

Acne, Anti-fungal, Balancing, Brightening, Exfoliating, Itchy Skin, Lightening, Moisturizing, Soothing

5–6 Tablespoons ground oatmeal

1 Tablespoon milk

Add water till mixture forms a thick paste. Apply to skin & leave on for 10-20 minutes then rinse off with luke warm water.

## OILY SKIN PAPAYA AND CLAY WHITENING MASK

Cleansing, Balancing, Blackheads, Brightening, Calming, Cooling, Moisturizing, Oily Skin, Repairing, Soothing, Tightening

2 Teaspoons of cosmetic clay

1 Teaspoon of aloe vera or aloe vera juice

2 Tablespoons papaya pulp

Mix clay together with juice to make a fine paste. Apply the mask to a clean face and neck, avoiding the eye and lip areas. Leave on for 15 minutes. Rinse off with lukewarm water.

## OILY SKIN PEACH MASK

Anti-aging, Cleansing, Healing, Mature Skin, Moisturizing, Repairing, Scarring

1 peach (peeled and mashed)

1 Teaspoon of olive oil

Mix ingredients together, apply to skin and leave for 15 minutes, then rinse off with warm water.

## OILY SKIN SAGE FACE MASK

Acne, Anti-aging, Anti-fungal, Anti-inflammatory, Anti-oxidant, Antibacterial, Antiseptic, Balancing, Brightening, Calming, Cellulite, Cleansing, Exfoliating, Lightening, Mature Skin, Moisturizing, Soothing, Wrinkles

10 drops lavender oil

5 drops bergamot oil

3 drops clary sage oil

3 Tablespoon white corn meal

3 Tablespoons almond meal (freshly ground raw almonds work best)

Add just enough rosewater or orange flower water to make a wet paste.

Massage the mixture onto your face in gentle circular motions, avoiding the eye area. Leave the mixture on for 5 to 15 minutes, then rinse off with warm water.

## OILY SKIN SWEET PEPPER MASK FOR OILY SKIN

Balancing, Cleansing, Exfoliating, Itchy Skin, Moisturizing, Soothing

2 Tablespoons red or yellow sweet pepper pulp

1 egg white

1 Tablespoon plain yogurt

1 Tablespoon ground oatmeal

Mix the ingredients together and apply to skin. Leave on for 10-20 minutes then rinse off with luke warm water.

## OILY SKIN WHITENING MASK

Anti-aging, Anti-inflammatory, Anti-oxidant, Calming, Cleansing, Exfoliating, Healing, Mature Skin, Moisturizing, Repairing, Scarring

3 Teaspoons of low fat cottage cheese.

4 Teaspoons of plain Yogurt (non sweetened)

Separate egg white from one egg and whip it till frothy

3 drops of Hydrogen Peroxide Solution or lemon juice

Mix the ingredients together and apply to skin. Leave on for no more than 10 minutes then rinse off with luke warm water.

## OILY SKIN YEAST MASK FOR ACNE AND OILY SKIN

Anti-aging, Anti-inflammatory, Discoloration.

1 Teaspoon of yeast dissolved in boiled water – wait until it reaches the consistency of Yogurt or thick cream then Add a few drops of lemon juice. Apply to face and remove with warm water when completely dry.

## OILY SKIN/BLACKHEADS OIL BLEND

Acne, Age Spots, Anti-aging, Anti-fungal, Anti-inflammatory, Anti-oxidant, Antibacterial, Antifungal, Antiseptic, Balancing, Brightening, Cellulite, Cleansing, Discoloration, Exfoliating, Healing, Itchy Skin, Lightening, Mature Skin, Moisturizing, Repairing, Scarring, Soothing, Tightening, Wrinkles


10 drops evening primrose oil

10 drops macadamia oil

4 drops orange oil

4 drops grapefruit oil

5 drops tea tree oil

Mix these oils together and massage into skin.


## OILY SKIN ORANGE AND GUAVA FULL FACIAL TREATMENT

Acne, Anti-aging, Anti-fungal, Anti-oxidant, Brightening, Cleansing, Discoloration, Exfoliating, Exfoliating , Lightening, Moisturizing, Oily Skin, Soothing, Tightening


1 ripe guava fruit

½ an orange

2 or 3 soft guava leaves (optional)

2 Teaspoons milk powder or oatmeal powder

½ Teaspoon sea salt (optional)

Cut and deseed guava then dice into small pieces.  Add the optional leaves and other ingredients.  Blend well in a blender or mortar and pestle. Apply mixture to you skin in a soft massaging motion. Leave on for 10 minutes then wash of with warm water. Repeat application for another 10 minutes best results.

## OILY SKIN PARSLEY & LEMON DRYING AND WHITENING TINCTURE

Acne, Lightening, Oily Skin, Red Veins, Stimulating, Tightening

Soak 1 Tablespoon crushed parsley leaves (or 3 drops parsley oil)

1 Teaspoon lemon juice

1 Tablespoon water

Strain parsley out of juice and apply with cotton pad to skin. Let it dry, after a few minutes remove with lukewarm water. Repeat once a week.

## PROTECTIVE COCOA BUTTER SKIN CREAM

Anti-aging, Cleansing, Mature Skin, Moisturizing

4 oz cocoa butter

4 oz jojoba oil

2 oz shaved beeswax

4 drops essential oil

Melt beeswax and Cocoa Butter in a double boiler until melted and stir in Jojoba Oil, and any essential oils you want to scent it with into mixture. Pour into a glass jar. Apply as desired.

## RED VEIN ACNE PARSLEY TREATMENT

Antibacterial, Antiseptic, Red Veins

1 Teaspoon crushed fresh parsley leaves or stems or 4 drops parsley oil

4 drops of lemon juice

Apply Parsley juice on its own or mixed with lemon to your face. Wait to dry then rinse off with lukewarm water.

## RED VEIN TREATMENT OIL

Anti-aging, Moisturizing, Red Veins

2 Tablespoons almond or wheatgerm oil (can add 5 drops avocado oil also)

21 drops parsley oil

5 drops carrot seed oil

11 drops geranium oil

4 drops cypress oil

## RED VEINS OIL BLEND 2

Anti-aging, Antibacterial, Cleansing, Healing, Mature Skin, Moisturizing, Red Veins, Repairing, Scarring

2 drops parsley oil

10 drops jojoba oil

10 drops olive oil

Mix these oils together and massage into skin.

## RED VEINS PARSLEY ALMOND OIL BLEND

Anti-aging, Antiseptic, Antibacterial, Moisturizing, Soothing

4 drops parsley oil

1 Tablespoon almond oil

Blend oils together and apply to affected areas with cotton ball or as a night treatment.

## REJUVENATING FACIAL CLEANSER

Anti-aging, Cleansing, Healing, Mature Skin, Moisturizing, Repairing, Scarring

3 Tablespoons flax seed oil

3 Tablespoons extra virgin olive oil

6 Tablespoons grapeseed oil

15 drops of your favorite essential oils – optional neroli, orange or bergamot for example

Blend oils together and apply to skin in a gentle massaging motion. Rinse off with warm water.

## REJUVENATING, BRIGHTENING CARROT SEED OIL AND CUCUMBER SKIN TREATMENT

Acne, Age Spots, Anti-aging, Anti-oxidant, Antibacterial, Antiseptic, Balancing, Brightening, Cellulite, Cooling, Dark Circles, Discoloration, Healing, Lightening, Mature Skin, Moisturizing, Puffiness, Scarring,

Tightening, Wrinkles

2 Tablespoons grapeseed oil

1 inch of fresh cucumber mashed or pureed

3 drops of carrot seed oil essential oil

Blend ingredients together and apply to skin. Leave on for 10 minutes then rinse off with warm water.

## REPAIRING APPLE AND HONEY MASK

Anti-aging, Anti-inflammatory, Anti-oxidant, Calming, Cleansing, Exfoliating, Healing, Mature Skin, Moisturizing, Repairing, Scarring

1 grated apple

2 Tablespoons honey

Blend the ingredients together and apply to skin. Leave on for 10-20 minutes then rinse off with luke warm water.

## REPAIRING HEALING SCARRING DAMAGED SKIN OIL BLEND

Acne, Age Spots, Anti-aging, Anti-inflammatory, Anti-oxidant, Antibacterial, Antiseptic, Balancing, Brightening, Calming, Cellulite, Cleansing, Discoloration, Healing, Itchy Skin, Lightening, Mature Skin, Moisturizing, Repairing, Scarring, Soothing, Wrinkles

24 drops apricot kernel oil

8 drops calendula oil

6 drops carrot seed oil

7 drops chamomile oil

4 drops geranium oil

5 drops neroli oil

10 drops olive oil

10 drops rosehip oil

5 drops borage (starflower) oil (optional)

Mix these oils together and massage into skin. Allow to absorb into your skin for a few minutes, then apply your favorite moisturizer or foundation.


## REPAIRING OIL BLEND

Acne, Age Spots, Anti-aging, Anti-fungal, Anti-inflammatory, Anti-oxidant, Antibacterial, Antiseptic, Balancing, Brightening, Calming, Cellulite, Cleansing, Discoloration, Healing, Itchy Skin, Lightening, Mature Skin, Moisturizing, Moisturizing Acne, Repairing, Repairing Oil, Scarring, Soothing


8 drops calendula oil

4 drops calophyllum oil

10 drops evening primrose oil

4 drops geranium

4 drops manuka oil

10 drops olive oil

10 drops jojoba oil

10 drops rosehip oil

Mix these oils together and massage into skin.

## REPAIRING PROTEIN FACIAL

Anti-aging, Anti-inflammatory, Anti-oxidant, Balancing, Calming, Cellulite, Cleansing, Exfoliating, Healing, Mature Skin, Moisturizing, Repairing, Scarring, Soothing

¼ cup barley or oat flour

1 Teaspoon brewer's yeast

2 Tablespoons honey

1 Vitamin E capsule

1 egg yolk (optional)

2 Tablespoon almond oil

¼ cup buttermilk or yogurt

Mix together to form a smooth paste. Apply to skin and leave on for 15-20 minutes before rinsing off with warm water.

## REPAIRING PUMPKIN Yogurt MASK

Acne, Age-spots, Anti-aging, Anti-fungal, Anti-inflammatory, Anti-oxidant, Brightening, Calming, Cleansing, Exfoliating, Healing, Lightening, Mature Skin, Moisturizing, Repairing, Scarring, Soothing

2 cups canned pumpkin

4 Tablespoons greek yogurt

4 Tablespoons honey

1 Teaspoon pumpkin pie spice

Mix the ingredients together and apply to skin. Leave on for 10-20 minutes then rinse off with luke warm water.

## REPAIRING YOGURT ALOE VERA MASK

Acne, Balancing, Calming, Cooling, Moisturizing, Repairing

½ cup of natural yogurt

2 Tablespoons aloe vera gel (or gel from inside the fresh aloe vera leaf)

Mix ingredients together and apply to face. Leave on for 15-30 minutes then rinse off with water.

## SCARRING REDUCTION SCAR REMOVING FACIAL OIL

Anti-fungal, Anti-inflammatory, Antibacterial, Antiseptic, Balancing, Calming, Cellulite, Cleansing, Healing, Repairing, Scarring, Soothing

1 oz calophyllum oil

15 drops galbunam oil

15 drops lavender oil

Blend oils together. Apply a little of this oil to your scars with a cotton ball or q-tip after washing your face. When skin has absorbed all the oil you can apply moisturizers or makeup. Used daily this will reduce the appearance of scars - newer scars will heal faster.

## SOOTHING ACNE RED WINE FACE MASK

Acne, Anti-aging, Anti-inflammatory, Anti-oxidant, Balancing, Calming, Cleansing, Cooling, Exfoliating, Healing, Mature Skin, Moisturizing, Repairing

2 Tablespoons red wine

½ Tablespoon aloe vera gel

1 Tablespoon organic Honey

1 Tablespoon kelp Powder – Seaweed powder

Mix the Honey and other ingredients together then leave it to rest for 10 minutes so the kelp powder can absorb the wet ingredients. Apply to face and leave on for around 10 minutes then wash off with warm water.


## SOOTHING BAKING SODA BODY SCRUB RECIPE

Age Spots, Anti-aging, Anti-inflammatory, Balancing, Cellulite, Cleansing, Itchy Skin, Mature Skin, Moisturizing, Soothing


1/3 cup baking soda

½ cup almond oil

½ Teaspoon of vitamin E

10 drops of fragrance or essential oil, optional

Mix ingredients together and apply to your skin with a gentle rubbing motion. Rinse off after you are finished scrubbing.


## STIMULATING ANTIOXIDANT BODY SCRUB

Brightening, Calming, Cleansing, Exfoliating, Healing, Lightening, Moisturizing

10 drops grapefruit oil, lemon oil or juice

1/4 cup olive oil

1/4 cup brown sugar

Mix ingredients together and apply to your skin with a gentle rubbing motion. Rinse off after you are finished scrubbing. Can also add oatmeal and adapt this scrub as you wish by adding fruit pulp or ground nuts and seeds.

## SOOTHING CALMING CHAMOMILE FOR SKIN LIGHTENING

Anti-aging, Anti-inflammatory, Anti-oxidant, Brightening, Calming, Cleansing, Exfoliating, Healing, Itchy Skin, Lightening, Mature Skin, Moisturizing, Repairing, Scarring, Soothing

3 Teaspoons of dried chamomile flowers or chamomile tea

1 Cup of water

1 Tablespoon honey

1 Tablespoon rose water

Pour one cup of water into a pan and bring to a boil. Add Chamomile and simmer for ten minutes (or use chamomile tea). Add other ingredients and allow to cool.

Apply solution with a cotton pad to your face and neck. Leave it on for 15 minutes, then rinse off with warm water. Use every other day. Store the solution in an airtight container for up to a week in the refrigerator.

## SOOTHING CLEANSING BANANA MINT MASK

Balancing, Cleansing, Exfoliating, Itchy Skin, Soothing, Tightening

1/4 cup instant oatmeal

1 small banana

1 egg white

1 mint tea bag

Mix the ingredients together and apply to skin. Leave on for 10-20 minutes then rinse off with luke warm water.

## SOOTHING ELDERFLOWER SKIN SOFTENING AND SUNBURN FACIAL TREATMENT

Anti-aging, Anti-inflammatory, Anti-oxidant, Balancing, Calming, Cellulite, Cleansing, Mature Skin, Moisturizing, Soothing, Soothing Moisturizing

1-2 cups elderflowers

½ cup almond oil

1 large jar

A pan of hot water

A piece of muslin/cheese cloth for straining the mixture or pantyhose.

Glass jars to store the formula in.

Place the muslin cloth or pantyhose in the jar so that the edges stretch or hang over the sides of the jar. Fill the muslin/pantyhose with elderflowers. Add just enough flowers to the Almond Oil so the flowers are covered. Stand the jar in a pan of boiling water and simmer for approx two hours or alternatively you can use a slow cooker with lid on and sit the jar inside with the jar top covered in cooking foil to prevent steam entering the mixture. Allow to cool until you can handle the cloth without burning your fingers. Squeeze the liquid into the jar. Discard the first flowers then Apply as desired with a cotton ball in a circular motion.

## SOOTHING GREEN TEA AND CHAMOMILE TEA TONER

Anti-oxidant, Brightening, Calming, Healing, Itchy Skin, Lightening, Scarring, Soothing

Make two cups of tea using green and chamomile tea bags. Spray onto skin or apply with a cotton pad. Leave on skin until dry then apply moisturizer.

## SOOTHING INFLAMED SKIN OIL BLEND

Acne, Anti-aging, Anti-fungal, Anti-inflammatory, Antibacterial, Antiseptic, Balancing, Calming, Cellulite, Cleansing, Healing, Insect Repellant, Itchy Skin, Mature Skin, Moisturizing, Repairing, Scarring, Soothing, SPF Protection

8 drops calendula oil

4 drops karanja oil

4 drops lavender oil

4 drops neem oil

20 drops olive oil

20 drops coconut oil

Mix these oils together and massage into skin.

## SOOTHING MOISTURIZING OATMEAL YOGURT MASK

Anti-aging, Anti-inflammatory, Anti-oxidant, Balancing, Calming, Cleansing, Exfoliating, Healing, Itchy Skin, Mature Skin, Moisturizing, Repairing, Scarring, Soothing

1 Tablespoon oatmeal finely ground

1 Tablespoon live, organic plain yogurt

¼ Teaspoon of honey

Mix the ingredients together and apply to skin. Leave on for 10-20 minutes then rinse off with luke warm water.


## SOOTHING OATMEAL AND BASIL MASK

Acne, Balancing, Cleansing, Itchy Skin, Soothing


2-3 Teaspoon of crushed basil leaves

1 Tablespoon oatmeal

Water to mix

Mix the ingredients together and apply to skin massaging in a circular motion. Leave on for 10-20 minutes then rinse off with luke warm water.


## SOOTHING OIL BLEND

Acne, Age Spots, Anti-aging, Anti-fungal, Anti-inflammatory, Anti-oxidant, Antibacterial, Antiseptic, Balancing, Brightening, Calming, Cellulite, Cleansing, Healing, Insect Repellant, Itchy Skin, Lightening, Mature Skin, Moisturizing, Repairing, Scarring, Soothing, Wrinkles


24 drops almond oil

8 drops calendula oil

4 drops calophyllum oil

7 drops chamomile oil

4 drops lavender oil

10 drops macadamia oil

10 drops wheat germ oil

15 drops safflower oil

5 drops neem oil

Mix these oils together and massage into skin.

## SOOTHING Sensitive Skin MASK

Balancing, Calming, Itchy Skin, Moisturizing, Soothing

This mask is great for soothing chapped, sunburned or irritated skin.

1 cup natural yogurt

½ cup oatmeal (ground)

You can also use egg white instead of Yogurt in this recipe for tightening and lightening skin.

Mix the ingredients together and apply to skin.  Leave on for 10-20 minutes then rinse off with luke warm water.

## SOOTHING YOGURT MASK (GREAT FOR A SUNBURNT OR WINDBURNT FACE)

Acne, Anti-aging, Anti-fungal, Anti-inflammatory, Anti-oxidant, Brightening, Calming, Cleansing, Exfoliating, Healing, Lightening, Mature Skin, Moisturizing, Repairing

1 Tablespoon natural yogurt, at room temperature

1 Teaspoon runny honey (use 2 Teaspoon for drier skin)

NATURAL HOME MADE SKIN CARE RECIPES

3 drops of fresh lime juice for oily skin

Mix the ingredients together and apply to skin. Leave on for 10-20 minutes then rinse off with luke warm water.


## SOOTHING ACNE UMF HONEY, TEA TREE, LAVENDER SPOT SERUM

Anti-fungal, Anti-aging, Anti-oxidant, Anti-inflammatory, Antiseptic, Brightening, Cleansing, Discoloration, Exfoliating, Moisturizing, Soothing


2 Tablespoons UMF honey

3 drops tea tree oil

3 drops lavender oil or rosemary oil

Blend together and apply to affected areas. Leave on for a few minutes then wash off with warm water or a cotton ball.


## STIMULATING ANISE STEAM FACIAL

Anti-bacterial, Stimulating


4 Cups water

1-3 drops anise seed oil

1/3 cups whole cloves

3-5 drops essential peppermint oil

Boil a kettle or pot full of water then add the herbs. Boil for a minute or two then remove from heat. Cover and let steep for 5 minutes. Place pot on dishcloth on counter or table and remove the lid.

Cover your head with a large, clean towel and position your face over the steaming water with the towel acting as a tent over the bowl to capture the steam. Keep your eyes closed and your face at least 10-12

167

inches from the boiling water during the facial. Enjoy the fragrance about 5-7 minutes. Once the facial is over, splash face with slightly cool water.

## STIMULATING ANTI-OXIDANT GINGER POMEGRANATE FACE MASK

Acne, Age Spots, Anti-inflammatory, Anti-oxidant, Balancing, Brightening, Cleansing, Discoloration, Exfoliating, Lightening, Repairing, Stimulating, Tightening

2 Tablespoons grated ginger root

3 Tablespoons pomegranate pulp or juice

Grate ginger and mix with enough pomegranate juice to create a smooth mixture.

Apply to face for 20 minutes, then rinse off with warm water.

## STIMULATING ANTIOXIDANT CITRUS OIL BLEND

Acne, Age Spots, Anti-aging, Anti-inflammatory, Anti-oxidant, Balancing, Brightening, Cellulite, Cleansing, Discoloration, Exfoliating, Healing, Lightening, Mature Skin, Moisturizing, Repairing, Scarring, Tightening

4 drops orange oil

3 drops lemon oil

10 drops jojoba oil

10 drops grape seed oil

Mix these oils together and massage into skin.

## STIMULATING COFFEE FACIAL MASK FOR CLEAR SKIN

Acne, Anti-fungal, Brightening, Exfoliating, Lightening, Moisturizing, Soothing, Stimulating

3 Tablespoons used finely ground coffee brewed in a little boiling water (can strain it through a coffee filter) or 1 strong shot of espresso coffee

1 small glass of milk

Mix ingredients together and apply the mixture to your skin. You can include the coffee grinds as an exfoliator also. Rinse off with warm water.

## STIMULATING OIL BLEND

Anti-aging, Cleansing, Moisturizing, Stimulating

3 drops anise seed oil

15 drops jojoba oil

10 drops grape seed oil

Mix these oils together and massage into skin.

## TIGHTENING AUTUMN APPLE FACIAL MASK

Acne, Anti-aging, Anti-inflammatory, Anti-oxidant, Balancing, Calming, Cleansing, Exfoliating, Healing, Itchy Skin, Mature Skin, Moisturizing, Repairing, Scarring, Soothing, Tightening

¼ of an apple cooked and mashed

1 Tablespoon honey

1 Tablespoon oatmeal

Mix ingredients together and apply to skin.  Leave on for 10 minutes then rinse off with warm water.

## TIGHTENING CEDARWOOD GERANIUM FACIAL SERUM

Anti-aging, Anti-inflammatory, Anti-oxidant, Balancing, Calming, Cleansing, Exfoliating, Healing, Mature Skin, Moisturizing, Repairing, Scarring

½ cup full fat organic yogurt

1 Teaspoon honey

1 drop cedarwood oil

1 drop geranium oil

Mix all  together until thoroughly blended.  Apply mixture to skin using fingertips and a gentle motion. Leave on for 10 minutes, rinse off with warm water.

## TIGHTENING EGG WHITE FACELIFT MASK

Anti-aging, Blackheads, Brightening, Cleansing, Exfoliating, Lightening, Moisturizing, Oily Skin, Tightening, Wrinkles

2 egg whites

1 Teaspoon of sugar or honey

Whisk the egg yolks until the mass is firm and consistent

Add Sugar, Cleansing, Exfoliating, Moisturizing gradually and mix well to combine the two

Apply on the face and leave on for 25 minutes

Wash off with warm water using a wash cloth

The use of albumin is well known among major cosmetics companies. The most popular, Mario Badescu's Temporary Lifting Mask uses albumin to immediately tightens, cleans and refines skin.


## TIGHTENING OIL BLEND

Acne, Anti-aging, Antifungal, Anti-inflammatory, Anti-oxidant, Antibacterial, Antiseptic, Balancing, Cellulite, Cleansing, Discoloration, Exfoliating, Healing, Mature Skin, Moisturizing, Soothing, Tightening


2 drops eucalyptus oil

4 drops tea tree oil

4 drops orange oil

20 drops jojoba oil

20 drops almond oil

Mix these oils together and massage into skin.


## TIGHTENING PORE MINIMIZING EGG WHITE MASK

Age spots, Anti-oxidant, Cleansing, Tightening


1 egg white whipped lightly

½ Teaspoon lemon juice

Slowly add lemon juice to egg white. Apply to face with cotton ball and allow to dry. Reapply another layer and allow that to dry.

Rinse off with warm water.

## TIGHTENING SKIN FIRMING FACIAL MASK

Anti-aging, Anti-inflammatory, Anti-oxidant, Calming, Cleansing, Exfoliating, Healing, Mature Skin, Moisturizing, Repairing, Scarring

1 Tablespoon honey

1 egg white

1 Teaspoon glycerin

Enough flour, arrowroot, oatmeal or chickpea flour to create a paste. Mix all ingredients together and apply to face leaving on for 10 minutes before rinsing off with warm water.

## TONERS

Apply by spritzing with a spray bottle or with a cotton pad & leave to dry before applying moisturizer.  Can also be used to steam your skin by adding to a steam vaporizer.

**Sensitive Skin:** Chamomile tea and/or a drop of chamomile oil in a cup of water or tea

**Acneic Skin:** 2 drops lavender oil, 2 drops rosemary oil, 1 drop tea tree oil in a cup of water

**Normal or Dry Skin:** 2 drops rose oil, 1 drop sandalwood oil, 1 drop palma rosa oil (optional) in a cup of water

**Normal or Oily Skin:** 2 drops orange oil (or lemon), 1 drop neroli oil, 2 drops chamomile oil or use 1 cup of chamomile tea instead of a cup of water for the whole recipe

## WRINKLE AVOCADO FACEMASK FOR DRY SKIN

Anti-aging, Anti-oxidant, Antibacterial, Antiseptic, Cleansing, Healing, Mature Skin, Moisturizing, Repairing, Scarring, Wrinkles

½ an avocado

1 Teaspoon almond meal or almond oil

1 Teaspoon jojoba or olive oil

Mix all ingredients together and apply to skin. Leave on for 15 minutes then rinse off with warm water.

## WRINKLE OIL BLEND

Anti-aging, Anti-oxidant, Antibacterial, Antiseptic, Balancing, Cleansing, Healing, Itchy Skin, Mature Skin, Moisturizing, Repairing, Scarring, Wrinkles

10 drops apricot kernel oil

10 drops avocado oil

10 drops borage oil

10 drops jojoba oil

3 drops clary sage oil

5 drops wheat germ oil

Mix these oils together and massage into skin.

## WRINKLE PREVENTATIVE

2 Tablespoon almond, wheatgerm or apricot kernel oil

2 drops chamomile oil

8 drops neroli oil

7 drops geranium oil

2 drops carrot seed oil

5 drops fennel oil

4 drops lavender oil

Blend together and store in a glass bottle out of sunlight. I prefer to store this in a dropper bottle so you can use it easily. Apply twice daily morning and night.

## WRINKLE SERUM FOR MATURE SKIN (OVER 50)

10 drops carrot seed oil

2 drops myrhh oil

10 drops carrot seed oil

10 drops rosehip oil

9 drops evening primrose oil

10 drops borage oil

5 drops galbanum oil

10 drops neroli oil

You can add 4 drops violet leaf oil as well but it's optional

Blend together and store in a glass bottle out of sunlight. I prefer to store this in a dropper bottle so you can use it easily. Apply twice daily morning and night.

## WRINKLE SERUM FOR OVER 30'S

2 Tablespoons almond, wheatgerm or apricot kernel oil

8 drops clary sage oil

10 drops palma rosa oil

9 drops yarrow oil

7 drops fennel oil

6 drops carrot seed oil

5 drops borage oil

6 drops jojoba oil

2 drops patchouli oil

8 drops rose oil

Blend together and store in a glass bottle out of sunlight. I prefer to store this in a dropper bottle so you can use it easily. Apply twice daily morning and night.


## WRINKLE SERUM FOR OVER 40'S

2 Tablespoons almond, wheatgerm or apricot kernel oil

9  drops neroli oil

9  drops lavender oil

9 drops fennel oil

10 drops frankincense oil

2 drops rosemary oil

9 drops evening primrose oil

8 drops borage oil

5 drops rosehip oil

3 drops lemon oil

10 drops carrot oil

Blend together and store in a glass bottle out of sunlight. I prefer to store this in a dropper bottle so you can use it easily. Apply twice daily morning and night.

## WRINKLE BUSTING CUCUMBER MAYO MASK

Age Spots, Anti-aging, Anti-oxidant, Antibacterial, Antiseptic, Balancing, Brightening, Cooling, Dark Circles, Discoloration, Lightening, Mature Skin, Moisturizing, Puffiness, Repairing, Tightening, Wrinkles

½ cucumber unpeeled and mashed or pureed

1 egg white

2 Tablespoons mayonnaise

½ cup oil wheat germ, olive or avocado oil

Wash the Cucumber but don't peel it, mix with other ingredients. Apply morning and evening, and gently wipe off with warm water or a cotton pad.

## WRINKLES EYE SERUM

Anti-aging, Anti-fungal, Anti-oxidant, Antibacterial, Antiseptic, Balancing, Calming, Cellulite, Cleansing, Mature Skin, Moisturizing, Soothing, Wrinkles

2 Tablespoons hazelnut oil

6 drops borage seed oil

9 drops evening primrose oil

6 drops lavender oil

6 drops carrot oil

2 capsule vitamin E

Mix these oils together and store in glass eye dropper jar. Shake well before each use.

Take one drop and gently apply to eye area before bedtime.


## WRINKLES CARROT HONEY MASK

Anti-aging, Anti-inflammatory, Anti-oxidant, Calming, Cleansing, Exfoliating, Healing, Mature Skin, Moisturizing, Repairing, Scarring


1 Tablespoon honey

1 Tablespoon carrot pulp or juice

Mix the ingredients together and apply to skin. Leave on for 10-20 minutes then rinse off with luke warm water.


You can mix and match the ingredients in these recipes to create your own custom made treatments.


Now that you know what different ingredients can be used for specific conditions you can enjoy creating your own specific recipes.


Don't be afraid of experimenting. You can store these recipes in the refrigerator or even the freezer for later use.

# CONCLUSION

Thank you for taking the time to read this book. I hope you have enjoyed the recipes and information I've shared with you.

Please feel free to visit www.naturalskincarerecipes.com for any questions or comments you have to share. You can also use our Recipe Wizards online to quickly find suitable ingredients for masks and treatments as well as oil blends.

Create your own oil recipe here with our Serum Wizard: http://www.naturaskincarerecipes.com/wiz

For all ingredient suggestions use the Ingredient Wizard:

http://www.naturaskincarerecipes.com/wiz2

Have a great day!

**Mia**

# INDEX

# B

# C

8143241R00101

Made in the USA
San Bernardino, CA
29 January 2014